D1153808

OXFORD MEDICAL PUBLICATIONS

Emergencies in Adult Nursing

Emergencies in Adult Nursing

Edited by

Philip Downing

Vice Chair
Faculty of Emergency Nursing;
Lead Nurse for Emergency Care
Gloucestershire Hospitals NHS Foundation Trust
UK

Editorial advisor

Mark Allan

Emergency Department Consultant
Gloucestershire Royal Hospital
UK

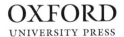

OXFORD
UNIVERSITY PRESS

OXFORD
UNIVERSITY PRESS

Great Clarendon Street, Oxford OX2 6DP

Oxford University Press is a department of the University of Oxford.
It furthers the University's objective of excellence in research, scholarship,
and education by publishing worldwide in

Oxford New York

Auckland Cape Town Dar es Salaam Hong Kong Karachi
Kuala Lumpur Madrid Melbourne Mexico City Nairobi
New Delhi Shanghai Taipei Toronto

With offices in

Argentina Austria Brazil Chile Czech Republic France Greece
Guatemala Hungary Italy Japan Poland Portugal Singapore
South Korea Switzerland Thailand Turkey Ukraine Vietnam

Oxford is a registered trade mark of Oxford University Press
in the UK and in certain other countries

Published in the United States
by Oxford University Press Inc., New York

British Library Cataloguing in Publication Data
Data available

Library of Congress Cataloging in Publication Data
Data available

Typeset by Cepha Imaging Private Ltd., Bangalore, India
Printed in China
on acid-free paper by
Asia Pacific Offset Limited

ISBN 978–0–19–922657–3

10 9 8 7 6 5 4 3 2 1

Preface

Nurses, in whatever environment they practice, may be faced with patients who develop sudden unexpected changes in their clinical condition. This handbook aims to assist nurses in assessing these potential emergency situations and guide them in their initial management.

The book utilizes a range of clinical presentations first developed by the Manchester Triage Group and since adopted as a national triage standard throughout the UK and beyond.

Each chapter identifies those presentations which are true emergencies requiring immediate intervention within seconds rather than minutes, those that are urgent and therefore need action within minutes rather than hours, those which need timely attention within minutes or hours, and those which are non-urgent and therefore are not time dependant. The key signs and symptoms, history and assessment, observations and findings, investigations, and actions and treatment are identified for each of the clinical conditions identified.

Philip Downing

Acknowledgements

I would like to thank all the contributors for the time and effort they have put into making the book a reality. I am indebted to all those colleagues who I have had the pleasure to work with over the years and who have been generous with their help and advice. I am also grateful to the team at OUP for their encouragement and patience during the writing of this book. Finally I would especially like to thank Lesley and Harriet for their support, patience, and understanding, and without whom the book would not have been possible.

Contents

Detailed contents

Contributors

Dr Mark Allan
Emergency Department Consultant
Gloucestershire Royal Hospital
Gloucestershire, UK

Ms Alison Ashley
Senior Sister
Cheltenham General Hospital
Gloucestershire, UK

Ms Sherri Cheal
Member of the Faculty of Emergency
Nursing and Deputy Lead Nurse for
Emergency Care
Gloucestershire Royal Hospital
Gloucestershire, UK

Ms Marilyn Gilbert
Senior Sister
Emergency Department
Cheltenham General Hospital
Gloucestershire, UK

Ms Jeanette Welsh
Fellow of the Faculty of Emergency
Nursing and Emergency Care
Practice Development Nurse
Emergency Department
Gloucestershire Royal Hospital
Gloucestershire, UK

Symbols and Abbreviations

📖	cross reference
>	greater than
<	less than
AAA	abdominal aortic aneurysm
ABG	arterial blood gas
AF	artrial fibrillation
AIDS	acquired immune deficiency syndrome
AMI	acute myocardial infarction
ATLS	Advanced Trauma Life Support
AV	arteriovenous
AXR	abdominal x-ray
βhCG	beta-human chorionic gonadotropin
BP	blood pressure
bpm	beats per minute
C&S	culture and sensitivity
CCU	coronary care unit
CN	cyanide
CO	carbon monoxide
CO_2	carbon dioxide
COHb	carboxyhaemoglobin
COPD	chronic obstructive pulmonary disease
COSHH	Control of Substances Hazardous to Health
CRP	C-reactive protein
CSF	cerebrospinal fluid
CT	computed tomography
CT-PA	computed tomography pulmonary angiogram
CVA	cerebral vascular accident
CVE	cerebral vascular event
CXR	chest x-ray
D&C	dilation and curettage
DKA	diabetic ketoacidosis
DPL	diagnostic peritoneal lavage
DSF(ab)	digoxin-specific Fab
DTs	delirium tremens
DVLA	Driver and Vehicle Licensing Agency
DVT	deep vein thrombosis

ECG	electrocardiogram
EDC	date of confinement
ENT	ear, nose, and throat
FB	foreign body
FBC	full blood count
G	gauge
GA	general anaesthetic
GCS	glucocorticosteroid or Glasgow Coma Score
GI	gastro-intestinal
GORD	gastro-oesophageal reflux disease
GP	general practitioner
GTN	glyceryl trinitrate
GUM	genitourinary medicine
Hb	haemoglobin
HDU	high dependency unit
HIV	human immunodeficiency virus
HRT	hormone replacement therapy
ICP	intracranial pressure
ICU	intensive care unit
IDDM	insulin-dependent diabetes mellitus
IM	intramuscular
IU	international units
IUD	intrauterine device
IV	intravenous
KUB	kidney, ureter, bladder
L	litre(s)
LFT	liver function test
LMP	last menstrual period
LOC	level of consciousness
LVF	left ventricular failure
m	metre
mcg	microgram
mg	milligram
MI	myocardial infarction
min	minute(s)
MRC	Medical Research Council
NAC	N-acetylcysteine
NG	nasogastric
NICE	National Institute for health and Clinical Excellence

NIDDM	non-insulin-dependent diabetes mellitus
NSAID	non-steroidal anti-inflammatory drug
O_2	oxygen
OCP	oral contraceptive pill
OPG	orthopantomogram
OTC	over-the-counter
$PaCO_2$	partial pressure of carbon dioxide in arterial blood
PCI	percutaneous coronary intervention
PE	pulmonary embolism
PEA	pulseless electrical activity
PEFR	peak expiratory flow rate
PHTLS	Pre-Hospital Trauma Life Support
PID	pelvic inflammatory disease
PPE	personal protective equipment
PQRST	palliative/provocative, quality, region/radiation, severity, timing
PR	per rectum
PROM	premature rupture of membranes
PV	vaginal bleeding
SAH	subarachnoid haemorrhage
SC	subcutaneous
sec	second(s)
SPF	sun protection factor
SpO_2	saturation of peripheral oxygen
STD	sexually transmitted disease
SVT	supraventricular tachycardia
TB	tuberculosis
TBSA	total body surface area
TCA	tricyclic antidepressant
TFT	thyroid function test
TIA	transient ischaemic attack
TMJ	temporomandibular joint
TNCC	Trauma Nursing Core Courses
TPR	temperature, pulse, and respirations
U&Es	urea and electrolytes
URTI	upper respiratory tract infection
UTI	urinary tract infection
V/Q	ventilation/perfusion
VF	ventricular fibrillation
VT	ventricular tachycardia
XR	X-ray

Chapter 1

Abdominal pain

Differential diagnosis

☼ True emergencies
- Aortic aneurysm
- Diabetic ketoacidosis
- Ectopic pregnancy
- Gastro-intestinal bleed
- Myocardial infarction
- Peritonitis

☼ Urgent presentations
- Appendicitis
- Cholecystitis
- Intestinal obstruction
- Pancreatitis
- Peptic ulceration
- Renal colic
- Sickle cell crisis
- Trauma
- Urinary retention

⑦ Non-urgent presentations
- Constipation
- Dysmenorrhoea
- Endometriosis
- Gastritis
- Gastroenteritis
- Hepatitis
- Hernia
- Irritable bowel syndrome
- Ovarian cyst
- Pelvic inflammatory disease
- Urinary tract infection

Introduction

Due to the number of organs within the abdominal cavity there are a wide variety of conditions which initially present with abdominal pain. Reducing the possibilities to a manageable number does not require formal abdominal examination in the first instance. A clear history of events and assessment of the patient along with their baseline clinical observations will usually make clear how ill the patient is. Beware, however, 'non-abdominal' conditions masquerading as abdominal pain. The prime culprits for this are ischaemic heart disease and diabetic ketoacidosis (DKA), both of which are life-threatening emergencies.

In all cases quickly survey the patient for obvious problems:

- Are they approximately the right weight for their height?
- What does the patient's face tell you—do they appear in pain? Are they distressed? Are they sweating?
- Is the patient bent over, splinting their abdomen, writhing, pacing, assuming a rigid position, changing position frequently, lying back, relaxed?
- Look at the skin: note colour, turgor, and integrity. Pallor, sweating, and cool, clammy skin indicate potential shock. Dry skin and mucous membranes suggest dehydration
- Temperature: pyrexia suggests inflammatory or infectious causes. Hypothermia suggests circulatory compromise
- Pulse: tachycardia will occur with shock, fever, pain, sepsis, or anxiety. A weak, rapid pulse suggests haemodynamic compromise
- Respiratory rate: depth and rate alter due to hypoxia, pain, or anxiety
- Blood pressure (BP): hypotension may indicate haemodynamic instability and must not be ignored. Hypertension can occur with myocardial ischaemia or anxiety
- Pregnancy testing: *must* be done in all female patients of child-bearing age. An ectopic pregnancy is a life-threatening emergency.
- Urinalysis: a negative test reduces the probability of a urinary tract infection (UTI)

The differential diagnoses have been listed by clinical urgency but remember that for a patient with abdominal pain the pain is the most dominant factor, regardless of the cause, and pain relief is their top priority.

☠ Aortic aneurysm

An abdominal aortic aneurysm (AAA) occurs following weakness in or damage to the wall of the aorta. This is often due to atherosclerosis.
The weakened wall may rupture and cause catastrophic blood loss. Aneurysms are most frequently found in the over 65 age group. Leaking or ruptured aneurysms carry a high mortality. The survival rates for emergency AAA surgery can be as low as 20%.

Key signs and symptoms
- Pain:
    - usually in the back, radiating to flank or groin
    - may be described as tearing or ripping
- Signs of hypovolaemia:
    - clammy
    - extreme pallor
    - breathlessness
    - cold
    - abdominal skin mottling
    - weak or absent pedal pulses
    - altered conscious level
    - collapse
- Pulsatile abdominal mass, tender on palpation may be present

Key history and assessment
- Middle aged or elderly patient
- Known AAA
- History of atherosclerosis
- Peripheral vascular disease
- Hypertension
- Cigarette smoker
- Hypercholesterolaemia.

Key observations and findings
- Pulse:
    - rate: tachycardia due to haemorrhage
    - thready quality
    - weak or absent femoral pulses
- Respiratory rate: tachypnoea
- Oxygen (O_2) saturation: may be difficult to record due to peripheral vasoconstriction
- BP: hypotension due to haemorrhage
- Delayed capillary refill
- Temperature: usually normal

Key investigations
- Continuous cardiac monitoring
- 12-lead electrocardiogram (ECG)
- Laboratory investigations:
    - arterial blood gases (ABGs)

- full blood count (FBC): looking specifically for haemoglobin (Hb) and platelet levels
- urea and electrolytes (U&Es)
- glucose: raised in stress
- cross-match at least 8 units
- Chest x-ray (CXR)
- Emergency portable abdominal ultrasound if available
- Abdominal CT scan may be considered if the patient is stable

Key actions and treatment
- Requires immediate medical assessment
- If the patient is critically ill, the diagnosis should be made clinically and the patient transferred for surgery without delay
- Undertake primary survey assessment
- High flow O_2 via a non-rebreathing mask
- Large-bore IV access in both arms, 14 gauge (G) cannula
- Intravenous (IV) morphine for pain relief, carefully titrated. Remember opiates can reduce conscious level and reduce BP
- Controlled fluid resuscitation with warmed fluid to bring systolic up to *no more* than 100mmHg. 0.9% saline in the first instance, then blood when available
- Catheterize: hourly measurements essential to monitor renal function and response to fluid resuscitation
- Calm and controlled manner: most patients are frightened and need to be reassured by competent professional staff
- Prepare for a fast but controlled transfer to theatre
- Ensure consent obtained if possible
- Prepare relatives for the possibility that surgery may have a poor prognosis

☠ Diabetic ketoacidosis

A presentation of widespread abdominal pain can be associated with diabetic ketoacidosis (DKA). The cause of this is not fully understood but it is thought to be related to the metabolic and electrolyte disturbance.

Any infective process raises the blood glucose as a response to stress. If the patient does not increase their insulin accordingly they may develop DKA as a result. A similar process may occur in patients with non-insulin-dependent diabetes mellitus (NIDDM).

To ensure DKA is not overlooked blood glucose levels should be checked on all patients with abdominal pain.

📖 See Diabetes, p.157.

☠ Ectopic pregnancy

This is the development of a fetus at a site other than in the uterus. The most common type occurs in a Fallopian tube. As the fetus grows the Fallopian tube will become blocked and rupture. The condition is likely to present in the first 6–8 weeks of pregnancy. A patient with an ectopic pregnancy will present with lower abdominal or suprapubic pain which worsens dramatically when rupture occurs. The patient may also have signs and symptoms of significant blood loss. Pregnancy testing will be positive and the patient may have a history of previous ectopic pregnancy.

📖 See Pregnancy, p.333.

☠ Gastro-intestinal bleed

Gastro-intestinal (GI) bleeds can occur from any site within the GI tract. Upper GI bleeds, from the stomach or duodenum, are the most common. Peptic ulceration accounts for >50% of GI bleeds and can present with epigastric pain. Any patient presenting with abdominal pain should have peptic ulceration and GI bleed excluded.

📖 See GI bleed, p.245.

☠ Myocardial infarction

Myocardial infarction (MI) can present with acute epigastric pain. Atypical presentations are more common in the elderly. A careful history is required to exclude MI and a 12-lead ECG recorded if there is any doubt.

📖 See Chest pain, p.115.

☣ Peritonitis

Inflammation of the peritoneum may be caused by bacteria carried in the bloodstream or, more commonly, perforation or rupture of the GI tract. Peritonitis is a serious condition which carries the risk of septicaemia.

Key signs and symptoms
- Pain: generalized and severe
- Difficulty breathing due to pain
- Clammy/sweaty
- Pallor
- Reluctant to move due to pain
- Abdomen rigid

Key history and assessment
- Recent symptoms of appendicitis
- Severe abdominal pain

Key observations and findings
- Pulse:
  - rate: tachycardia due to haemorrhage or sepsis
  - weak or thready quality
- Respiratory rate: tachypnoea due to haemorrhage or sepsis
- O_2 saturation: may be difficult to record
- BP: hypotensive due to internal haemorrhage
- Temperature: may be high with infection or low in severe sepsis

Key investigations
- Laboratory investigations:
  - ABG
  - FBC
  - U&E
  - glucose: raised in stress.
  - group and hold, cross-match if signs of blood loss

Key actions and treatment
- Requires immediate medical assessment
- High-flow O_2 via a non-rebreathing mask
- Wide-bore IV access in both arms
- IV morphine for pain relief, carefully titrated, as opiates will reduce respiratory rate and BP
- IV anti-emetic if nausea or vomiting present
- Early IV antibiotics according to local protocols
- Nil orally
- Nasogastric (NG) tube
- Fluid resuscitation: use saline in the first instance
- Catheterize: hourly measurements essential to monitor renal function and response to fluid resuscitation
- Calm and controlled manner: most patients are frightened and need to be reassured by competent professional staff
- Prepare for an urgent but controlled transfer to theatre

✪ Appendicitis

Inflammation of the appendix. This is usually acute and if not treated by appendicectomy can progress to cause an abscess or peritonitis.

Key signs and symptoms
- Pain: classically starts as a mild central abdominal pain for 6–12 hours before localizing to the right Iliac fossa
- Rebound tenderness and guarding on palpation may be present
- Atypical presentations are common
- Nausea
- Vomiting
- Loss of appetite
- Mild pyrexia
- Hunched over to relieve tension of abdominal wall (curl up into fetal position when lying down)

Key history and assessment
- Commonest in ages 8–25 years, but can occur in all age groups
- Gradual increase in pain and pyrexia over preceding 48 hours
- Anorexia

Key observations and findings
- Pulse: rate—may have a tachycardia due to pain
- Respiratory rate: may have a tachypnoea due to pain
- O_2 saturation: usually normal
- BP: usually normal
- Temperature: usually mild pyrexia 38°C

Key investigations
- Laboratory investigations:
  - FBC: looking specifically for raised white cell count
  - U&E
  - glucose: raised in stress

Key actions and treatment
- Requires urgent medical assessment
- Wide-bore IV access in one arm
- IV morphine for pain relief, carefully titrated, as opiates will reduce respiratory rate and BP
- IV anti-emetic if nausea and vomiting (N&V) present
- IV saline to maintain hydration
- Nil-by-mouth
- Calm and controlled manner: most patients are frightened and need to be reassured by competent professional staff
- Prepare for a timely transfer to surgical ward or theatre

☼ Cholecystitis

Inflammation of the gall bladder, often caused by blockage of the bile duct with gall stones. This condition is potentially serious and may result in septicaemia or peritonitis.

Key signs and symptoms

- Pain in right upper quadrant and epigastrium: sometimes referred to tip of right shoulder
- Pallor
- Nausea
- Vomiting
- Possibly some degree of jaundice—check sclera first
- Pyrexia

Key history and assessment

- History/family history of gallstones
- >40 years old
- More common in women than men
- More common in overweight patients

Key observations and findings

- Pulse: rate—may be tachycardia due to pain or sepsis
- Respiratory rate: may be tachypnoea due to pain or sepsis
- O_2 saturation: usually normal
- BP: hypotension may occur if sepsis present
- Temperature: usually pyrexial

Key investigations

- Laboratory investigations:
  - FBC: baseline only
  - U&Es
  - liver function tests (LFTs)
  - glucose: potentially raised due to stress
  - serum amylase to exclude pancreatitis, which may also be caused by gallstones

Key actions and treatment

- Requires timely surgical assessment
- IV access
- IV morphine for pain relief, carefully titrated to patient's perception of pain relief and clinical observations, as opiates will reduce respiratory rate and BP
- IV anti-emetic if required
- IV fluid—on hydration maintenance regimen.
- IV antibiotics according to local protocol
- Transfer to a surgical ward

:✪: Intestinal obstruction

Obstructions can occur in either the large or small bowel and may result from:
- Adhesions from previous surgery
- Faecal impaction
- Gallstones
- Tumours
- Hernias

Key signs and symptoms
- Abdominal pain
- Nausea
- Vomiting, may be faeculent or contain partially digested food according to the level of the obstruction
- Constipation
- Small amounts of diarrhoea

Key history and assessment
- History of previous surgery
- Known gallstones
- Known hernia
- Previous severe constipation
- Recent unintended weight loss

Key observations and findings
- Pulse: rate—may have tachycardia due to pain
- Respiratory rate: may be tachypnoea due to pain
- O_2 saturation: usually normal
- BP: usually normal, but may be lowered or elevated
- Temperature: usually normal

Key investigations
- Laboratory investigations:
  - FBC
  - U&E
  - glucose: raised in stress
- Abdominal XR (AXR): to confirm diagnosis of obstruction

Key actions and treatment
- Requires urgent surgical assessment
- IV access
- IV morphine for pain relief, carefully titrated, as opiates will reduce respiratory rate and BP
- IV fluid on hydration maintenance regimen
- Nil-by-mouth
- NG tube
- Anti-emetic drugs are ineffective and therefore contraindicated
- Transfer to surgical ward

:✪: Pancreatitis

Inflammation of the pancreas can be acute, chronic, or relapsing and may be associated with gallstones or alcoholism. The pancreatic duct becomes blocked, preventing the release of pancreatic enzymes into the small bowel. The enzymes continue to be produced and cause inflammation of the pancreas. In the chronic phase it may lead to malabsorption syndromes and diabetes.

Key signs and symptoms
- Abdominal pain:
  - upper left quadrant and epigastrium
  - may be referred to back and left shoulder
- Nausea
- Vomiting

Key history and assessment
- History of alcoholism
- Known gallstones
- Recent unintended weight loss

Key observations and findings
- Pulse: rate—may have tachycardia due to pain
- Respiratory rate: may have tachypnoea due to pain
- O_2 saturation: usually normal
- BP: usually normal—may be hypotensive due to malabsorption and severe pain responses
- Temperature: may be normal or slightly raised
- Capillary blood glucose: essential to check whether condition is affecting glucose control

Key investigations
- Laboratory investigations:
  - FBC
  - U&E
  - glucose: need to compare to capillary blood glucose, double-checking potential diabetes as a result of pancreatitis
  - amylase: may need to request separately from U&E in some labs. A high amylase, usually over 1000IU is diagnostic

Key actions and treatment
- Requires urgent surgical assessment
- IV access
- IV morphine for pain relief, carefully titrated, as opiates will reduce respiratory rate and BP
- IV anti-emetic if nausea or vomiting is present
- IV fluid on hydration maintenance regimen in the first instance
- Nil-by-mouth
- Position patient according to their comfort—should be able to lie straighter once adequate pain relief provided
- Transfer to surgical ward

☼ Peptic ulceration

Ulceration of the mucosal lining may occur in the stomach (gastric ulcer) or upper small intestine (duodenal ulcer). Major complications of ulcers include bleeding and perforation; peptic ulceration is the commonest cause of haematemesis and melaena. Historically believed to be a stress related condition it is now known that infection with the bacteria, *Helicobacter pylori* is the commonest cause. Other causative or aggravating factors include smoking, excessive alcohol and overuse of certain drugs (especially non-steroidal anti-inflammatory drugs (NSAIDs)). Less commonly ulceration may result from Crohn's disease or stomach cancer.

Key signs and symptoms
- Excessive belching
- Pain:
  - often described as heartburn, indigestion, or dyspepsia
  - ranges from nagging discomfort, to sharp and severe or burning sensation
  - upper, central abdominal pain (epigastric); does not normally radiate
  - related to eating—gastric ulceration pain worsens after food, duodenal ulceration pain relieved by eating
  - relieved by antacids
  - beware cardiac pain may mimic dyspepsia
- Nausea and retching
- Haematemesis
- Melaena
- Anaemia due to chronic low-grade bleeding
- Sudden onset of severe epigastric pain, spreading across the abdomen and rigidity of the abdomen may indicate perforation

Key history and assessment
- Exclude myocardial ischaemia
- Diagnosis based on history of symptoms and relationship of pain to eating and drinking
- Assessment of lifestyle, alcohol consumption, use of tobacco, weight, use of NSAIDs

Key observations and findings
- Temperature, pulse, BP
- Any abnormalities may indicate bleeding or perforation and should trigger further medical assessment

Key investigations
- FBC for anaemia
- Group and hold/cross match (if bleeding is evident)
- Erect CXR if perforation suspected: may reveal free air under the diaphragm
- In non-emergency situations investigations can be organized in primary care. These may include a breath or blood test for *H. pylori*

Key actions and treatments

- Haematemesis:
  - immediate medical support
  - maintain airway and breathing
  - ensure patent airway
  - remove blood/vomitus with a wide-bore suction catheter
  - O_2 administered via non-rebreathing mask at 15L
  - emergency anaesthetic assessment if reduced Glasgow Coma Score (GCS) or patient requiring urgent transfer to theatre
  - IV access with a wide-bore cannula $\times$ 2
  - IV fluids and blood transfusion according to local guidelines/medical advice
  - medical/surgical referral according to local protocol
  - catheterization and hourly monitoring for fluid balance control
  - provide clear explanation to patients
- Urgent referral to surgeons if suspected perforation:
  - IV access
  - IV analgesia
  - nil orally
  - IV fluids to maintain BP but do not over infuse as there is a risk of bleeding
- Non-emergency presentations:
  - simple over-the-counter (OTC) antacids may be tried
  - histamine (H2)-antagonists, such as ranitidine or cimetidine
  - advise to avoid food and drinks which trigger symptoms, stop smoking, stop using NSAIDs
  - refer to primary care for further investigation and management

☼ **Renal colic**

The development of stones in the kidney or ureter can lead to the sudden onset of severe pain. It is more common in men than women and occurs most commonly between the ages of 35–45.

Key signs and symptoms
- Pain:
  - unilateral loin or flank pain, depending on the location of the stone
  - radiating to the groin, thigh, or genitalia
  - may move if the stone moves
- N&V
- Urinary symptoms: haematuria may be present
- Sweating
- Restlessness due to colicky nature of pain

Key history and assessment
- Previous renal colic
- Recent dehydration—the condition is commoner in warm climates

Key observations and findings
- Pulse: may be tachycardic due to pain
- BP: may be hypertensive due to pain
- Temperature: apyrexial, unless accompanying infection
- Respiratory rate: normal unless affected by pain
- Normal SpO_2

Key investigations
- Urinalysis: the presence of blood on bedside urinalysis increases the likelihood of the diagnosis
- Urine for microscopy and culture
- Kidney, ureter, bladder (KUB) XR is of little value as although 90% of stones are radio-opaque, they are usually too small to visualize on a plain film
- CT is the definitive test
- Bloods for FBC, U&E, creatinine, calcium, phosphate, and urate

Key actions and treatment
- Pain relief is paramount
- Intramuscular NSAID, diclofenac 75mg intramuscularly (IM) or 150mg per rectum (PR)
- If unable to use NSAID then morphine or diamorphine IV, titrated to the patient's response, should be used
- An anti-emetic may be required
- Antispasmodics have not been demonstrated to have any benefit
- Encourage fluid intake
- Monitor urine output to ensure no obstruction
- Admit surgical ward if pain is not controlled or CT scan demonstrates evidence of blockage

:⚙: Sickle cell crisis

Sickle cell disease is a hereditary blood disorder that affects people with Black-African or Mediterranean ancestry. There is a lesser incidence in people of Asian ancestry. It is characterized by the production of abnormal Hb. The red blood cells are distorted into a characteristic sickle shape when blood O_2 levels are low. The distorted cells are rapidly removed from the circulation, causing anaemia. In crisis the sickle-shaped cells 'stack' on top of each other blocking a blood vessel. This causes widespread, severe pain. Resolution of the crisis requires fluid resuscitation and oxygenation. Beware of crises occurring in pregnancy as components of the treatment will adversely affect the fetus.

Key signs and symptoms
- Severe generalized pain, may affect abdomen
- Nausea
- Vomiting

Key history and assessment
- History of sickle cell disease ± crisis
- Family history of sickle cell disease

Key observations and findings
- Pulse: may have tachycardia due to pain and anaemia
- Respiratory rate: may have tachypnoea due to pain and anaemia
- O_2 saturation: <94%
- BP: usually normal or high due to pain
- Temperature: usually slightly pyrexial

Key investigations
- Laboratory investigations:
  - FBC: looking specifically for low Hb
  - U&E
  - glucose: raised in stress

Key actions and treatment
- Regular, known sickle cell patients may have an individualized management plan. A copy of this should be available to staff. These patients can withstand very large doses of opiates and will often require an analgesia infusion
- Requires urgent medical assessment
- Require high-flow O_2 therapy via a non-rebreathing mask
- IV access
- IV morphine for pain relief, carefully titrated to patient's perception of pain relief and clinical observations, as opiates will reduce respiratory rate and BP
- IV fluid: usually 0.9% saline
- Transfer to a haematology/medical ward

⊕ Trauma

Both blunt and penetrating trauma can affect the abdomen. Damage is caused by a variety of mechanisms of injury such as road traffic collisions, assaults, falls, or sporting injuries. Any abdominal organ may be involved, with the liver and spleen being most commonly injured. The main problems which arise are haemorrhage and organ laceration or perforation. Haemorrhage can be occult and the effects take a while before the patient demonstrates clinical features. Perforation of the bowel will result in spillage of the contents into the abdominal cavity and result in infection and peritonitis. Abdominal pain is present/with to a greater or lesser extent of all these injuries. The key is to determine which patients have pain solely due to abdominal muscular strains and which have underlying serious pathology.

📖 See Major trauma, p.293.

⊕ Urinary retention

The inability to pass urine causes severe lower abdominal pain. The enlarged bladder is often visible and is normally easily palpated unless the patient is very obese. Pain or the urge to urinate is increased on palpation. The patient gives a history of inability to urinate.

📖 See Urinary problems, p.421.

⑦ Non-urgent conditions

Even though the following conditions are clinically non-urgent, remember that the patient is in pain and may be frightened about what is happening. It is important to remember that conditions which at first may appear to be minor such as a UTI can become serious if not treated early.

⑦ Constipation

Faeces are hard and small, and defaecation causes difficulty or pain. Constipation can cause intestinal obstruction. Recurrent and long-standing constipation should be managed by Primary Care Services.

⑦ Dysmenorrhoea

Painful menstruation. The pain may start before or with menstruation and there are a variety of causes, including pelvic inflammatory disease (PID), endometriosis, fibroids, and the presence of an intrauterine device (IUD).

⑦ Endometriosis

This is a major cause of chronic abdominal pain in women. The pain is caused by uterine tissue being deposited in areas other than the uterus. These may then bleed at menstruation causing severe pain. This rarely requires admission as an emergency, but does need investigation and follow-up by gynaecology.

⑦ Gastritis

Gastritis is a term used to describe a number of conditions which inflame the lining of the stomach. It can be caused by infection with *H. pylori*, excessive alcohol intake, or prolonged use of NSAIDs. Gastritis can also occur after severe trauma, especially burns, serious infection, or major surgery. The most common presentation is abdominal pain which is described as burning, but may be felt as a tightness or heaviness. There is a relationship to food, with light meals often relieving the pain, and alcohol or caffeine making it worse. Symptoms may be relived with antacids. Associated symptoms include excessive belching and an uncomfortable feeling of fullness. The condition can be accompanied by N&V. *There is a risk that cardiac pain can be mistaken for gastritis and this should always be borne in mind.* A 12-lead ECG should be recorded in all cases.

⑦ Gastroenteritis

Most people at some time will experience gastroenteritis. It is normally a viral infection, although it can be caused by bacteria or parasites. The patient may experience abdominal pain accompanied by diarrhoea, vomiting, or both. Most cases resolve without medical intervention.

📖 See Diarrhoea and vomiting, p.163.

⑦ Hepatitis

Inflammation of the liver, usually caused by viruses, toxic substances, or immunological abnormalities. The condition may cause jaundice and right upper quadrant abdominal pain. Hepatitis B and C are blood-borne and can be contracted from the patient if a sharps injury occurs. Be sure to use personal protective equipment correctly, observing universal precautions and following local policies.

⑦ Hernia

The protrusion of an organ or tissues out of its usual body cavity. The usual reason for emergency presentation is severe pain because the hernia has become strangulated. In this case treat as for intestinal obstruction.

⑦ Irritable bowel syndrome

A common condition of unknown aetiology in which there is recurrent abdominal pain with constipation and diarrhoea at unpredictable intervals. This can continue for years without any deterioration in the patient's overall health, but it is a major restrictor of lifestyle.

⑦ Ovarian cyst

Fluid-filled sacs, which develop on one or both ovaries. More than one can develop at the same time. They can reach a very large size, twist, and cut off the blood supply causing severe ischaemic pain, which requires urgent surgery. More usually patients need referral to gynaecology as an outpatient for elective removal at a future date.

⑦ Pelvic inflammatory disease

Can be an acute or chronic condition in which the uterus, fallopian tubes, and ovaries are inflamed and infected. The infection may spread from an adjacent infected organ e.g. appendix, or it may result from a sexually transmitted infection, most commonly chlamydia. PID is a major cause of female infertility due to blockage of the fallopian tubes. It is characterized by lower abdominal pain, which can be severe. Referral to gynaecology is required.

⑦ Urinary tract infection

Cystitis and pyelitis can both cause lower abdominal pain or loin pain. The signs and symptoms vary with age, sex, and location of the infection.

📖 See Urinary problems, p.421.

Chapter 2

Abscesses and local infection

Differential diagnosis

☺ True emergencies

- Epiglottitis
- Gas gangrene
- Necrotizing fasciitis

☼ Urgent presentations

- Osteomyelitis
- Septic arthritis

ⓘ Timely assessment

- Cellulitis
- Dental abscesses
- Soft tissue infections

☠ Epiglottitis

A localized bacterial infection, usually caused by *Haemophilus influenzae B*, or streptococci. The infection causes swelling of the epiglottis, increasing dysphagia, stridor, and swelling of the larynx. It is a life-threatening emergency due to the resultant airway obstruction.

Do not examine the mouth or throat due to the risk of causing laryngeal spasm and airway obstruction.

📖 See Sore throat, p.391.

☠ Gas gangrene

Death and decay of wound tissue infected by the soil bacterium *Clostridium perfringens*. The toxin produced by the bacterium causes putrefactive decay of connective tissue with the generation of gas. Incubation can be as little as 1 hour but more commonly is 1–4 days post injury.

Key signs and symptoms

- Sudden onset of severe pain at wound site
- Discolouration of skin
- Weakness and tiredness
- Offensive smelling wound
- Surgical emphysema in tissues surrounding wound
- Delirium
- Visible necrotic tissue

Key history and assessment

- Traumatic wound in contaminated conditions e.g. farm machinery

Key observations and findings

- Pulse: tachycardia
- Respiratory rate: tachypnoeic
- BP: hypotension
- Capillary refill delayed
- O_2 saturations: initially normal, may drop <94%
- Temperature: low grade pyrexia

Key investigations

- ABGs: if any respiratory distress or signs of hypoxia
- FBC: raised white cell count is usual
- U&Es: baseline for renal function
- Glucose: may be elevated

Key actions and treatment

- Requires early surgical assessment
- 100% O_2 via a non-rebreathing mask
- Large bore IV access: 14G cannulae
- Immediate IV antibiotics: in line with local guidelines
- Fluid resuscitation:
  - monitor fluid balance
  - catheterize and monitor hourly
- IV pain management
- Anticipate early transfer to high dependency unit (HDU) or for surgery
- Psychological care of patient and family
- Report case to health protection agency
- Hyperbaric O_2 therapy may be required as O_2 inhibits bacterial growth

☢ **Necrotizing fasciitis**

Infection affecting the fascia surrounding the muscles as well as limb tissue and the abdominal wall. It is caused by the bacteria *Streptococcus pyogenes*. It usually affects people who are already immunocompromised following damage to the skin or long-term IV drug abusers. Prompt treatment does not guarantee survival, or that patients who do survive will not require amputations.

Key signs and symptoms
- Pain which is excessive in relation to, or at a site distant to, the injury
- Diarrhoea and vomiting
- Weakness, muscle pain, excessive tiredness
- Dehydration and oliguria
- Pus-filled blisters which may bleed
- Gangrene
- Delirium

Key history and assessment
- Diagnosis based on signs and symptoms
- Immunocompromised patients
- Traumatic wound in contaminated conditions

Key observations and findings
- Pulse: tachycardia
- Respiratory rate: tachypnoeic
- BP: hypotension, may be profound
- Capillary refill delayed, often only seen in younger patients
- O_2 saturations, initially normal, may drop <94%

Key investigations
- Blood tests should not delay diagnosis and treatment
- ABGs: if any respiratory distress or signs of hypoxia
- FBC: raised white cell count is common
- U&Es: baseline for renal function
- Glucose

Key actions and treatment
- Requires early surgical assessment
- 100% O_2 via a non re-breathing mask
- Large bore IV access: 14G cannulae
- May require early placement of central line to facilitate IV access
- Immediate IV antibiotics
- Aggressive fluid resuscitation
  - monitor fluid balance
  - catheterize and monitor hourly
- IV pain relief as required
- Anticipate need for immediate aggressive surgery to debride gangrenous tissue
- Psychological support to patients and family
- Report case to health protection agency

⚙ Osteomyelitis

Infection within bone, which may follow an open fracture or be caused by blood-borne organisms. If untreated it can lead to abscess formation within the bone, non union of fractures, or septicaemia.

Key signs and symptoms
- Pain over site on palpation or pressure
- Local inflammation
- Slow or non-healing wound to affected part

Key history and assessment
- Compound, or possibly open, fracture in previous few weeks
- Inoculation injury in previous few weeks

Key observations and findings
- Observations likely to be within normal limits
- May have low-grade pyrexia

Key investigations
- XR of affected part: positive finding = bone will have a 'fluffy' appearance. These findings often only occur after 5–7 days of illness and early false negatives are common and must be taken into consideration
- FBC: raised white cell count is usual
- U&Es: baseline for renal function
- Glucose: may be elevated
- Blood for culture and sensitivity (C&S)

Key actions and treatment
- Requires orthopaedic assessment
- IV access
- Early IV antibiotics
- Pain relief as appropriate
- Anticipate orthopaedic admission
- Stress to the patient the importance of staying in hospital as the condition can quickly become chronic and intractable
- May require surgery to drain any abscesses

:⚙: Septic arthritis

Infection within a joint space can be caused by many bacteria with *Staphylococcus aureus* being the most common. The knee is the most common site, although it can affect any joint.

Key signs and symptoms
- Intensely painful joint
- Hot, red, swollen joint
- Fever
- Reduced movement due to pain
- Joint held in flexion

Key history and assessment
- Joint penetration:
  - unintentional—wound
  - deliberate—joint aspiration, injection, surgery
- Steroid therapy

Key observations and findings
- Temperature: pyrexia
- Pulse: may have tachycardia due to infection
- BP: usually normal
- Respiratory rate: usually normal, but may be tachypnoeic if sepsis present

Key investigations
- XR of the joint: may be normal in the early stages
- FBC, blood glucose
- Blood for C&S
- Joint aspiration for C&S: *prior to antibiotic therapy*

Key actions and treatment
- Pain relief
- Antipyretic
- IV antibiotics, usually started with flucloxacillin
- Rest and elevation of the joint involved
- Refer to orthopaedics for admission

ⓘ **Cellulitis**

Inflammation of the dermis and SC tissues commonly due to bacterial infection with either streptococci or staphylococci which enter via a wound or damaged skin.

Key signs and symptoms
- Pain at the site of the infection
- Redness and swelling, initially at the wound or infection site, but then spreading
- Skin warm to touch
- Red tracking visible along limbs
- Localized lymph node enlargement
- Leakage of serous fluid or pus from skin
- Generally unwell, muscle pain, weakness and lethargy

Key history and assessment
- Possible wound (including puncture wounds) in previous few days
- Locally swollen: usually distal limbs

Key observations and findings
- Temperature: anticipate pyrexia, higher in more severe infections
- Pulse: possible tachycardia in response to pyrexia
- BP: usually normal
- Respiratory rate: usually normal
- Look for 'tracking': a red line leading away from the affected area towards the trunk, following line of lymph vessels
- Check for swollen lymph nodes at the junction of the affected limb and the trunk
- Pain score: likely to be mild-to-moderate
- Comparative measurements of both limbs at affected level

Key investigations
- Blood glucose
- May require FBC in more serious cases

Key actions and treatment
- Mark limits of redness with a ballpoint pen or permanent marker
- Mark limits of any tracking
- Oral antibiotics may be prescribed where there is no tracking and no joint involvement
- Analgesia as appropriate for the patient
- Antipyrexials as required
- Increase fluid intake
- Patients should be reviewed in unscheduled or primary care within 24 hours to ensure area of redness has not increased and that no tracking has developed
- Admit for IV antibiotics if any tracking present or suspicion of joint involvement

⚠ Dental abscesses

These are extremely painful and patients are usually 'at the end of their tether' with the pain. With an infection developing in a tooth as a result of decay or injury, formation of pus occurs under the tooth placing pressure on the nerve.

📖 See Dental problems, p.151.

ⓘ Soft tissue infections

A wide variety of soft tissue infections are routinely seen and treated in a wide range of care environments. Although non-urgent they cause considerable pain and distress to patients and should not be treated as trivial. In all cases it will be necessary to stress the importance of personal hygiene and the need to take action to prevent infection spread. Antibiotics are often, but not always, required. Incision and drainage of some abscesses may be undertaken by GPs or Emergency Department medical staff, but others will need admission.

Key signs and symptoms
- Pain: throbbing pain keeping the patient awake at night
- Mild pyrexia
- Localized heat, redness, pain, and swelling

Key history and assessment
- Establish exact location and description of infected area
- Does the pain keep the patient awake at night?
- Any recent trauma?
- Previous infections?
- Any systemic infections? Check for pyrexia
- Response to antibiotics, if any have already been given
- Consider diabetes especially:
  - if recurrent problem
  - combined with excessive thirst, tiredness, polyuria
- IV drug user, higher risk of developing soft tissue infections

Key observations and findings
- Observations usually within normal limits
- Check temperature
- Check capillary blood glucose: this will be raised in diabetics with infections

Key investigations
- Glucose may be requested if bedside glucose higher than normal
- C&S of pus if present

Key actions and treatment
Abscesses
A collection of pus enclosed by damaged and inflamed tissues. Found in a variety of areas on the body. Those within the skin will be 'ripe' for incision and drainage, either in an Emergency Department, general practice, or by a general surgeon, or the abscess will not have come to a head. In the latter case antibiotics may be required. Incision and drainage may be more complex than expected, with irrigation required to ensure the complete removal of all pus and careful wound dressing to prevent excessive bleeding, while encouraging drainage to prevent reformation. Analgesia is required until the infection has subsided.

Bartholin's cyst

An abscess or cyst can form in the Bartholin's glands, which are situated at the junction of the vagina and vulva. Their secretions normally lubricate the vulva to assist penetration by the penis during intercourse. Cysts or abscesses of these glands are very painful and the patient will find walking difficult, constrictive clothing uncomfortable, and an inability to sit down. Referral to gynaecology is required.

Boils

A boil is an abscess formed in the base of a hair follicle. Management is the same as for abscesses.

Breast abscess

Usually present as painful breast 'lumps'. Patients require oral antibiotics, aspiration of the abscess, and referral to a breast surgeon for follow-up. A high level of anxiety often accompanies breast abscesses and needs sensitive management.

Cysts

Abnormal sacs, lined with epithelium, filled with liquid or pus. They can occur anywhere on the body, but the generic term usually refers to cysts under the skin. These are easily excised and this can be done by the GP or in day surgery. If infected, a course of antibiotics should be prescribed.

Ear infections

These are extremely painful and all complaints of pain should be treated sympathetically. Patients require strong analgesia and should be advised how to combine paracetamol/codeine mixtures with NSAIDs. They should not go swimming or fly whilst the infection persists. Evidence suggests that the use of antibiotics in otitis media is of little benefit.

📖 See Ear problems, p.169.

Eye infections (bacterial)

Very common and usually treated with chloramphenicol, provided nothing more serious is found on thorough examination. Patients need to be shown how to bathe their eyes with warm water and cotton wool, how to use the chloramphenicol (including frequency and when to stop using it) and the importance of scrupulous hygiene.

📖 See Eye problems, p.183.

Foreign body (FB)

Any ignored FB can become infected. Management of FBs will depend on the object involved, its location, how long it has been in situ, and the general health of the patient. In the hand, anything other than the most superficial FB needs referral to an experienced practitioner.

📖 See Foreign bodies, p.233.

Glandular fever

Caused by the Epstein–Barr virus and affecting lymph nodes in the neck, armpits, and groin, mostly in adolescents and young adults. The lymph nodes will be swollen and tender, patients have a pyrexia, headache, sore throat, and loss of appetite. A monospot test should be undertaken.

Diagnosis is confirmed by a large number of monocytes in a differential white cell count. Beware development of meningitis symptoms, but otherwise patients should be advised to rest, not work, take simple analgesia, and plenty of fluids.

Gout

Caused by the deposition of uric acid crystals in joints and is most commonly seen in the fingers, toes, ears, and nose. Most patients will already have been diagnosed by their GP and already be on allopurinol, if not, refer to primary care. Otherwise advise simple analgesia during an attack and to book a review with their GP.

Herpes virus infections

Presents as cold sores, chicken pox, and shingles. Cold sores require treatment with OTC preparations. Chickenpox should be treated symptomatically and the patient kept away from work, school, and socializing until scabs have formed—usually 14 days. Patients should avoid all contact with pregnant women and newborn babies. Shingles usually affects older adults and is extremely painful. Analgesia needs to be thought out properly and referral to primary care for review is prudent. It may require additional treatment depending on the dermatome affected. Be extra careful where any part of the head is involved.

Impetigo

A highly contagious skin infection, usually caused by staphylococci. It can spread very quickly from an initial patch. Classically the small pustules join together to form crusty yellow sores. Scrupulous personal hygiene is vital—patients should not share towels and other wash items with other family members. Systemic antibiotics may be prescribed in some cases and topical in others.

Infected insect bites

A wide range of insect bites may become infected. It is important to distinguish between a normal inflammatory reaction and a developing infection. Usually 1% hydrocortisone cream is sufficient in the early stages, or systemic antibiotics if the patient is generally unwell with the bites. Consider if a localized infection may lead to a more generalized systemic problem.

📖 See Bites and stings, p.89.

Paronychia

An abscess of the nail fold which requires incision and drainage.

Perineal abscess

May occur on an episiotomy wound or be a peri-anal abscess. Both are very painful and need surgical assessment.

Pilonidal sinus

A short tract leading from an opening in the skin to the cleft at the top of the buttocks and containing hairs. These may be one-off or recurrent, but need surgical assessment.

Sexually transmitted diseases (STDs)

Policies for the management of patients with sexually transmitted diseases vary. Some genitourinary medicine (GUM) clinics prefer to see all suspected STDs and do not want unscheduled care areas to take swabs or prescribe antibiotics. Others will want swabs taken only, while some will want swabs taken and antibiotics commenced. It will be necessary to establish a local policy.

Upper respiratory tract infection (URTI)

Extremely common, particularly in those <5 or >75 years due to anatomical differences and inadequate immune systems. Generally antibiotics are only required for those with underlying respiratory disease or where chest examination is indicative of a chest infection. Otherwise patients should be advised to use paracetamol, steam inhalations, and OTC remedies for sore throats, rhinitis, and blocked sinuses.

📖 See Sore throat, p.391.

Wound infection

📖 See Wounds, p.427.

Allergy

Differential diagnosis

☉ True emergency
- Anaphylaxis

① Timely assessment
- Moderate allergic reaction

② Non-urgent presentation
- Localized allergic reactions

☠ Anaphylaxis

The general definition of anaphylaxis is an abnormal reaction to a particular antigen. In clinical practice 'anaphylaxis' is usually shorthand for 'anaphylactic shock', which is an extreme and generalized allergic reaction in which widespread histamine release causes swelling and constriction of the airways, circulatory collapse, and sometimes death.

Histamine release causes swelling of the soft tissues. The more widespread these symptoms, the more urgent the situation. The soft tissues of the face may be involved as may the soft tissue in the neck, mouth, and throat. Swelling in these areas can place the airway at risk from obstruction. Erythema and pruritus (itching) are common. The terms 'urticaria' or 'hives' refers to raised, erythematous, itchy lesions which can occur anywhere on the body. Angioedema usually occurs to the larynx, lips, eyelids, hands, feet, and genitals and results from involvement of the deeper dermal layers of the skin. Pruritus is uncommon in angioedema.

If the lower airways are affected the patient will present with an expiratory wheeze; upper airway involvement will result in inspiratory stridor. Vascular collapse occurs because histamine makes the capillaries 'leaky' and therefore fluid is lost into the tissue beds. This reduces the circulating volume causing hypotension and tachycardia. Abdominal cramps, vomiting, diarrhoea, and abdominal distension can occur, usually in response to an ingested allergen.

Anaphylaxis can be treated with drugs and judicious use of IV fluids. Some patients start with minor symptoms, which become more severe without treatment. At the other end of the scale some patients will develop anaphylactic shock with minimal warning. Patients with a history of previous anaphylaxis or those thought to be at high risk may carry an auto injector of adrenaline (epinephrine), such as an EpiPen® or Anapen®, which they can self-administer at the onset of an attack.

There is the potential for a secondary reaction up to 12 hours following the initial episode (a so-called biphasic reaction). This is usually less severe than the initial reaction. Patients should be advised to re-attend should symptoms return.

Key signs and symptoms
- Rash
- Itching
- Whole-body erythematous flushing
- Breathlessness
- N&V
- Abdominal pain
- Diarrhoea
- Stridor
- Laryngeal oedema
- Cyanosed
- Angioedema
- Airway obstruction
- Altered conscious level, agitation, confusion
- Collapsed and unconscious

Key history and assessment
- Known allergies
- Previous history of allergic reactions
- History of recent antigen exposure
- Family history of allergies, asthma, or eczema

Key observations and findings
- Pulse:
  - rate: commonly tachycardia
  - weak or thready pulse
- Respiratory rate:
  - tachypnoea
  - dyspnoea
- O_2 saturation: <94%
- BP: hypotension
- Continuous cardiac monitoring

Key investigations
- Treatment should be instigated before investigation
- Laboratory investigations:
  - ABGs: if any respiratory distress or signs of hypoxia
  - blood glucose

Key actions and treatment
- Requires immediate medical assessment
- Will require resuscitation facilities
- High-dose O_2 via a non-rebreathing mask
- IV access
- Observe for potentially life-threatening arrhythmias
- Pulse oximetry
- Remove causal agent if possible—e.g. bee sting
- IM adrenaline (epinephrine) 0.5mL 1:1000, can be repeated after 5min if required
- Antihistamine: IM chlorphenamine 10mg. Can be given slow IV
- Corticosteroid: IM hydrocortisone 200mg. Can be given slow IV in severe cases
- Adrenaline can be given IV if the patient is in shock.
  Continuous cardiac monitoring must be undertaken and the user *must* be experienced in managing the potential arrhythmias. *It must be in a dilution of at least 1:100,000*
- IV fluids
- Nebulized salbutamol
- In severe cases early ICU opinion will be required
- Calm and controlled manner: most patients are frightened and need to be reassured by competent professional staff
- Patient may also need:
  - IV ranitidine 50mg in 20mL saline over 10min to improve urticaria
  - IM glucagon if no progress being made and patient is on beta-blockers

① Moderate allergic reactions

Key signs and symptoms
- Rash
- Itching
- Widespread erythematous flushing

Key history and assessment
- Known allergies
- Previous history of allergic reactions
- History of recent antigen exposure
- Family history of allergies, asthma, or eczema

Key observations and findings
- Pulse: normal-to-mild tachycardia
- Respiratory rate: normal-to-mild tachypnoea
- BP: normal
- Pulse oximetry: should be normal

Key investigations
- None necessary for emergency treatment
- May require investigations later as an outpatient to determine causative agent

Key actions and treatment
- Requires early medical assessment
- High-dose O_2 via a non-rebreathing mask
- Full multi-parameter monitoring
- Remove causal agent, if possible—e.g. bee sting
- Oral chlorphenamine 4mg
- Observe for 1 hour
- If good response, discharge with 2 days' supply of chlorpheniramine
- If poor response move to guidelines for moderate anaphylaxis, see Anaphylaxis, p.32.

⑦ Localized allergic reactions

Whilst these are irritating to the patient they pose no danger and can be managed in primary care or at home using OTC medication. Examples include allergic conjunctivitis (hay fever).

Key signs and symptoms
- Pruritus
- Rhinitis
- Conjunctivitis

Key history and assessment
- Known allergies
- Previous history of allergic reactions
- History of recent antigen exposure
- Family history of allergies, asthma, or eczema

Key observations and findings
- Pulse: normal
- Respiratory rate: normal
- BP: normal

Key investigations
- None necessary for emergency treatment
- May have several investigations later as an outpatient to determine causative agent

Key actions and treatment
- Remove causal agent, if possible—e.g. bee sting
- Oral chlorpheniramine 4mg
- Observe for 1 hour
- If good response discharge with 2 days supply of chlorpheniramine and advise consultation with a pharmacist over suitable nasal spray
- If poor response move to guidelines for moderate anaphylaxis, 📖 see Anaphylaxis, p.32.

Further reading

Resuscitation Council (UK) (2005). *The Emergency Medical Treatment of Anaphylactic Reactions for First Medical Responders and for Community Nurses.* London: Resuscitation Council.

Apparently drunk

Differential diagnosis

:○: **Urgent presentation**
- Apparently drunk

① **Timely assessment**
- Alcohol ingestion

☼ Apparently drunk

Drinking of alcohol is common throughout the world. Acceptable levels of drinking, drinking habits, and the culture surrounding alcohol varies in different countries and within different societal groups. Government guidelines in the United Kingdom advise men not to regularly drink more than 3–4 units of alcohol per day or a total of 21 units in a week. Women should not regularly drink more than 2–3 units of alcohol per day or a total of 14 units per week. At least two alcohol-free days a week are recommended. A unit of alcohol is 8g of pure alcohol. The number of units of alcohol in common drinks are:

- 3 units:
  - pint of strong lager
  - pint of best bitter
  - pint of strong cider
- 2 units:
  - pint of ordinary strength lager
  - pint of ordinary bitter
  - pint of ordinary strength cider
  - 175ml glass of wine
- 1.5 units: alcopops
- 1 unit: pub measure of spirits

The majority of people are able to enjoy alcohol without any detrimental effects to their health. However, it is estimated that 1.8 million deaths occur worldwide each year as result of alcohol consumption. For people with a dependency on alcohol sudden withdrawal can cause severe physical and mental health problems.

Tempting as it is to dismiss anyone who smells strongly of alcohol as being 'just drunk'; this is a certain way to make a serious clinical error. Even with well-known patients, do not assume because they often fall over after drinking, that is what happened on this occasion. They may be intoxicated but may also be suffering from:

- Hypothermia
- Hypoglycemia
- Cerebral bleed
- Dehydration
- Head injury
- Self-harm
- Ingestion of other toxic substances

Many areas have an alcometer. This needs to be used with caution and patient consent must be obtained. Knowing that a patient has even a small amount of alcohol in their system does not obviate the necessity of excluding injury or illness. The greatest value of an alcometer is to facilitate psychiatric evaluation, as it is possible to demonstrate that a patient is not under the influence of alcohol and therefore fit for assessment.

⚠ Alcohol ingestion

If dealing with people under the influence of alcohol is a regular occurrence within your practice, consideration should be given to developing joint protocols with the local ambulance service and the local police service. This will ensure a consistent and safe approach to the management of these people and prevent front-line staff having to make difficult decisions in trying circumstances.

For patients who present to emergency care providers with problems as a result of alcohol, follow-up arrangements should be made with health education services or substance misuse teams. Referral protocols need to be established to ensure appropriate support is available. For patients not receptive to health advice at the time of presentation, strategies such as the placing of advice cards in pockets, follow-up with leaflets sent to their home address, or referral to their GP may be utilized.

Key signs and symptoms

- Smell of alcohol on breath
- Loss of inhibitions and inappropriate behaviour
- Altered conscious level:
  - dizziness and unsteady gait
  - ataxia
  - speech slurred
  - drowsiness
  - memory loss and confusion
  - Deterioration in conscious level
- Aggressive behaviour
- Incontinent of urine and sometimes faeces
- Vomiting

Be aware that alcohol absorption can continue for up to 2 hours following the last drink. The patient who is calming down may be experiencing a lowering of their conscious level to life-threatening levels.

Key history and assessment

- Clear denial of:
  - fall
  - diabetes
  - epilepsy
  - substance misuse
  - mental health problems
- Witness confirmation of alcohol intake
- Amount of alcohol drunk, over what period, any other substances taken?
- Any vomiting?
- Any potential injuries: has the patient fallen or been assaulted?
- Pre-existing medical problems, particularly diabetes
- Exclude hypoglycaemia, head injury, hypoxia
- Assessing the amount of alcohol consumed is often difficult

The acronym CAGE can be used to help assess if a patient is having a problem with alcohol consumption.

- have you ever felt the need to **C**ut down your alcohol intake?
- have you ever felt **A**nnoyed by people criticising you drinking?
- have you ever felt **G**uilty about the amount you drink?
- have you ever felt the need for an **E**ye opener in the morning?

A positive answer to 2 or more questions is suggestive of an alcohol problem.

Key observations and findings

- Frequent monitoring of vital signs required
- Pulse usually normal
- BP: may be low
- Respiratory rate, may be depressed in severe intoxication
- SpO_2, should be normal: further assessment required if <94%
- Temperature: ensure not hypothermic
- GCS: will require medical reassessment if decreasing

Key investigations

- 12-lead ECG:
  - if pulse is irregular
  - any report of chest pain
  - history of cardiac disease
  - any history of blackout, collapse, or loss of consciousness
- XR: if any report of trauma
- Laboratory investigations:
  - blood glucose
  - ABGs: if any respiratory distress or signs of hypoxia

Key actions and treatment

- Do not dismiss the patient as drunk. A patient with a reduced level of consciousness will have airway management problems regardless of the cause
- Establish and maintain a patent airway
- Beware of risk of aspiration of vomit
- Early medical assessment
- Protect from injury
- Consider removal of the patient's clothing:
  - 'drunks' are often incontinent of urine as they warm up
  - early removal of clothes ensures they have dry garments ready for discharge
  - maintain body temperature, do not allow them to become cold
- Encourage oral fluids and food if able to tolerate
- Anticipate admission if patient is unlikely to 'come round' in <4 hours
- Consider the need to treat thiamine (vitamin B1) deficiency
- Remain alert for a missed diagnosis
- Discharge only when able to protect own airway and when accompanied with a responsible adult who will stay with them until sober

Beware patients who may have ingested antifreeze (ethylene glycol)—they appear intoxicated and have sweet smelling breath. This is a medical emergency and requires urgent medical assessment.

Further reading

Kennedy J and Faugier J (1989). *Drug and Alcohol Dependency Nursing*. Oxford: Heinemann Nursing.

Assault

Differential diagnosis

☼ Urgent presentations

- Assault
- Domestic violence
- Non-accidental injury
- Sexual assault and rape

:O: Assault

Legally, an assault is committed whenever a threat is made upon a person. Battery is committed when a person is touched without their consent. There is no legal difference regarding the level of violence used to achieve assault or battery or in the level of harm caused for an individual to be charged with these crimes. Most victims of assaults are single young men, on low income, between the ages of 16–30 who have been drinking.

Key signs and symptoms
- The injuries incurred as a result of assault may be blunt or penetrating and affect any part of the body. In almost all cases there will be wounds
- Most commonly injuries are to the head, face, hands, and arms

Key history and assessment
- This is an area of healthcare that will potentially involve the police, lawyers, and the courts. Therefore all documentation relating to such cases must scrupulously adhere to the professional guidance on record keeping
- Assault is always 'alleged', as healthcare staff are rarely witnesses to the actual assault
- If the patient's words are used, these must be in quotation marks. All accounts must adhere to 'the patient reports that . . .' and clinical observations

Key observations and findings
- Varies according to the injuries sustained

Key investigations
- These will vary according to the nature and severity of the injury
- Local policies will differ, but as a general rule any breath, blood, urine, or other bodily samples required for evidence, rather than for clinical treatment, must be obtained by the police or by the police surgeon, with the explicit consent of both the patient and the treating clinician
- It is in the interests of everyone concerned that no profession is obstructed in carrying out their part of the process
- Clinical need takes priority over all other considerations
- The patient has the right to refuse any or all procedures, after they have had the purpose and benefit of those procedures explained
- It is wise to ensure that police photographers take any photographs required for evidential purposes, as photographs taken by clinical staff are rarely considered adequate evidence in court.

Key actions and treatments
- Where clothing is removed from the patient, great care must be taken not to disturb potential forensic evidence and therefore cutting of clothing should be kept to an absolute minimum, as this creates additional clothing fibres
- Where cutting is essential it is vital that this is not done through stab wound or bullet wound holes as this destroys evidence
- The officer concerned must sign for any clothes taken by police and each individual item must be put into brown-paper evidence bags.

Local police stations are usually more than happy to ensure that departments have an adequate supply of these
- Weapons that have been used in an assault must be retained for evidence, put into a police evidence bag, and labelled with the patient's name and date of alleged assault
- The minimum number of people should handle weapons and all those who do handle the item should do so wearing examination gloves
- Ideally the names of all those who handled the item should be listed on the evidence bag
- Confidentiality can and must be broken if firearms or knives are found as these constitute a threat to public safety and the police must be informed
- If a knife is still in the patient the only safe place for this to be removed is in theatre
- Under no circumstances should any clinical staff or police attempt to remove weapons from wounds until an experienced clinician has reviewed the patient
- Nurses should expect a police officer to be present with any such patient at all times until the weapon is handed to the officer. This is an essential part of the chain of evidence required in court
- Information about how to access further support if required

☼ Domestic violence

There is evidence to indicate that 1 in 4 women aged 16–59 and 1 in 7 men have been physically assaulted by their current or former partner. It is further estimated that 1 in every 10 heterosexual relationships and 1 in every 5 same-sex relationships involves physical abuse. In the UK one woman dies every week as a result of physical abuse by her partner. On average physical harm occurs 17 times before a victim seeks medical help.

Staff should be alert to a variety of presentations, from obvious injuries to repeated attempts at overdose or other forms of self-harm which may be associated with domestic abuse.

Whilst the decision to do anything about the abuse lies with the victim alone, healthcare staff must clearly establish the safety of any children living with the victim, their partner, or the couple. There is a clear link between domestic violence and child abuse and whilst an adult can make their own decision to report the abuse or not, there is a legal duty to protect children. Therefore whenever domestic violence is detected a referral to a paediatric liaison health visitor or social services must be initiated.

Key signs and symptoms
- Over-attentive or aggressive partner
- Patient withdrawn and reluctant to discuss events
- Injuries of a variety of ages evident
- Patient showing clear signs of fear
- Patient indicating that they do not expect to be believed
- Human bites
- Burns where the pattern or distribution suggest assault

Key history and assessment
- Presence and safety of children
- History not consistent with injury
- Delay in seeking treatment
- Incorporate a question about domestic violence into routine history taking, such as 'Has anyone ever physically hurt you?' Patients can then answer yes or no and choose to elaborate if a pause is left before moving on to the next question

Key observations and findings
- Injuries of varying ages present
- Defensive wounds to forearms

Key investigations
- Those relevant to presenting injury

Key actions and treatments
- Try to provide a secure environment where the victim can talk freely without fear of being overheard
- Document everything clearly and accurately, so that if the victim does decide to press charges then factually correct statements can be made

- Document suspicions of domestic violence, whether or not the victim concedes that this was the case
- Maintain a non-judgemental approach and resist the temptation to 'rescue' the victim
- Provide information on local domestic violence support organizations and helplines, explaining how they operate, and the safeguards used to protect victims. Men may need reassurance that such services are not only for women
- Indicate that the patient is not the only person to experience domestic violence, but that most people hide it. Abusers generally try to put the blame for the abuse on the victim and undermine their self-confidence and esteem, so do not expect a patient to be easily swayed from that belief
- Where the assault is considered to be serious, life-threatening, or there is a perceived risk to the public the police must be informed regardless of the patient's wishes. Otherwise referral must only be made with the patient's consent
- Refer all children in the relationship to a liaison health visitor or social worker

☼ Non-accidental injury

This applies to all vulnerable people but is generally applied to children. However, adults, especially the elderly, those with learning difficulties, chronic illnesses, or mental heath problems are also at risk. Some family court judges believe the term 'injuries not properly accounted for' is more accurate and helpful.

Abuse is defined as the act of harm to a person by a parent/relative/sibling/ other carer, either as a direct act or by a failure to provide proper care or protection, or both. Legal proceedings take place where there is evidence that suspicions are correct.

Healthcare staff are required to act as advocates for the vulnerable and should act on any suspicions. Abuse may take the form of:
- Physical abuse
- Emotional abuse
- Neglect
- Sexual abuse
- Financial abuse

In most cases the abuser in known to the patient and is in a position of trust.

Key signs and symptoms
- Patient very watchful of accompanying carer
- Disagreement of events between patient and carer
- Wounds in varying stages of healing
- Burns where the pattern or distribution suggest assault
- Poor hygiene suggesting neglect
- Injuries to the mouth or face
- Signs of restraint
- Dehydration or malnutrition

Key history and assessment
- Delay in presentation
- Multiple attendances
- Inappropriate or inconsistent history
- Obscure comments made by patient and dismissed by carer
- Incorporate a question into routine history-taking, such as 'Has anyone ever tried to hurt you?' leave the patient to answer as fully as they choose

Key observations and findings
- Injuries of varying ages present
- Poor rapport between vulnerable adult and accompanying carer
- Reluctance to answer questions without approval from carer

Key investigations
- Those relevant to presenting injury

Key actions and treatments

- Try to provide a secure environment where the victim can talk freely without fear of being overheard
- Document everything clearly and accurately, so that if the victim does decide to press charges then factually correct statements can be made
- Document suspicions of non-accidental injury, whether or not the victim concedes that this was the case
- Maintain a non-judgemental approach and resist the temptation to 'rescue' the victim
- Provide information on local social services and helplines, explaining how they operate and the safeguards used to protect victims
- Refer the patient to police or social services when they explicitly ask for this and when care homes or care staff are involved

✛ Sexual assault and rape

This is a terrifying and degrading experience for victims. In the majority of cases the attacker is known to the victim and may well be a partner, a relative, a friend, a workmate, or a neighbour. Ideally the patient should be seen and examined in a police rape suite by a police surgeon as soon as possible after the assault. This maximizes the chance of high-quality forensic evidence being obtained and thus a higher chance of a conviction in court. However, there are many reports of women feeling further degraded when this procedure is followed and therefore some victims will prefer to present to Emergency Care. These patients need time and great sensitivity.

If the victim has children and the assailant has access to the family then referral to a paediatric liaison health visitor or social services must be initiated in order to ensure the children's safety.

Key signs and symptoms
- Physical injury does not have to be present for sexual assault to have taken place
- A wide range of physical injuries may be present
- Patient may show signs of distress or may appear withdrawn

Key history and assessment
- Consideration needs to be given as to the best person to ask questions of the patient. Medical history relating to the extent of injuries may be asked by a healthcare professional, in the presence of a police officer if necessary. If the patient is medically stable, then questions relating to the incident are more appropriately asked by trained police officers
- Is the patient over 16—i.e. was it statutory rape?
- Date, time, and place of assault
- Any witnesses?
- What actually happened?
- Did penetration take place? If so, was this of the vagina, anus, or both?
- Did the perpetrator ejaculate? If so, was this into the vagina, anus, or onto clothing?
- Did the perpetrator use a condom?
- Were physical threats made?
- If female, what contraception method is the patient currently using, if any?
- If female, date of last menstrual period (LMP)?

Key observations and findings
- Injuries related to the mechanism of injury

Key investigations
- Urine for urinalysis and HCG
- All other investigations should be performed by a police surgeon to ensure quality of evidence

Key actions and treatments
- Medical resuscitation and treatment must take priority

- Care should be taken to preserve physical evidence wherever possible
- If the patient is medically stable then a purpose-designed rape suite may be the most appropriate place for assessment and treatment, if available. If not try to provide a secure environment where the victim can talk freely without fear of being overheard. Document everything clearly and accurately, so that if the victim does decide to press charges then factually correct statements can be made. Document claims and suspicions of sexual assault or rape, whether or not the victim concedes that this was the case
- Maintain a non-judgemental approach
- Consider the need for post exposure prophylaxis for HIV prevention
- Provide information on local rape crisis support organizations and helplines, explaining how they operate and the safeguards used to protect victims. Men may need reassurance that such services are not only for women
- Refer the patient to police or rape crisis team only when they explicitly ask for this
- Refer the patient to the GUM clinic for follow-up of potential STD
- Discussions should take place with local police services to formulate an agreement as to the reporting of serious sexual assaults whilst maintaining the victim's anonymity from the police if they wish not to report the crime themselves

Asthma

Differential diagnosis

☹ **True emergency**
- Life-threatening asthma

☼ **Urgent presentation**
- Severe asthma

① **Timely assessment**
- Moderate asthma

⑦ **Non-urgent presentation**
- Mild asthma

Introduction

Asthma is a chronic disease of the airways, which is characterized by acute exacerbations of wheezing. Typically the bronchial tree is inflamed and hyper-responsive to stimuli. In some patients a specific allergen is identified and a diagnosis of 'allergic asthma' can be made. Where an allergen cannot be identified the asthma is said to be 'idiopathic'. This includes asthma in response to exercise, NSAIDs, and environmental conditions. Bronchoconstriction results in chest tightness, dyspnoea, coughing, and expiratory wheeze. Often, but not always, the symptoms worsen at night. The British Thoracic Society and Scottish Intercollegiate Guidelines Network have produced a national clinical guideline for the management of asthma.[1]

☠ Life-threatening asthma

Key signs and symptoms

- Peak expiratory flow rate (PEFR) <33% predicted for age and gender or, more importantly, the patient's own normal reading
- Silent chest
- Cyanosis
- Feeble respiratory effort
- Unable to talk
- Exhaustion
- Confusion
- Coma

Key history and assessment

- Known asthmatic
- Previous admissions to an ICU due to asthma
- Previous hospital admissions due to asthma
- Chest pain: suggesting a complication such as a pneumothorax
- Usual medication: particularly note whether this includes steroids or theophylline
- Duration of symptoms: particularly wheeze, breathlessness, and nocturnal cough
- Onset of symptoms within minutes, rather than a deterioration over days or weeks
- Family history of atopic problems
- Smoker or living with a smoker
- Medication taken since attack started and its effectiveness

Key observations and findings

- Pulse: rate bradycardia or tachycardia
- Respiratory rate: bradypnoea <10bpm
- O_2 saturation:
  - <95% on O_2
  - <90% on air

- BP: hypotensive
- Continuous cardiac monitoring
- Temperature: pyrexia indicates infective cause, but otherwise will be normal
- PEFR: <33% predicted value

Key investigations
- CXR: may be requested if pneumothorax suspected
- Laboratory investigations: ABGs

Key actions and treatment
- Calm approach, as any sign of staff becoming excitable will exacerbate the feeling of rising panic already being experienced by the patient
- Immediate senior medical assessment
- 15L/min O_2 on non-rebreathing mask
- IV access
- Drug therapy
  - 5mg salbutamol nebulized on O_2. Repeat PEFR 15–30min after nebulizer
  - IV hydrocortisone 100mg
  - If no improvement within 15min:
    —repeat salbutamol nebulizer and add ipratropium bromide (Atrovent®) 0.5mg nebulizer
  - If no improvement within 30min:
    —may need aminophylline infusion (5mg/kg over 20min, followed by maintenance infusion of 0.5mg/kg/hour). Alternatively a salbutamol infusion 250mcg IV over 10min followed by a maintenance infusion may be considered
    —consider magnesium sulphate 2g IV over 30min
- Pneumothorax should be excluded
- Urgent ICU opinion may be required if the patient fails to improve or deteriorates

Further reading

1. BTS/SIGN (2008). British guideline on the management of asthma. A national clinical guideline. *Thorax*, **63**(supppl. iv), iv1–121 (doi:10.1136/thx.2008.097741) Available at : 🖳 http://www.sign.ac.uk/pdf/sign101.pdf

☼ Severe asthma

Key signs and symptoms
- PEFR: 33–50% predicted value based on age and gender or, more importantly, the patient's own normal reading
- Unable to talk in full sentences
- Respiratory rate: >25bpm
- Tachycardia: >110bpm
- Feeling of rising panic

Key history and assessment
- Known asthmatic
- Previous admissions to ICU due to asthma
- Onset of symptoms within minutes, rather than a deterioration over days or weeks
- Family history of atopic problems
- Exposure to known stimuli
- Chest pain: suggesting a complication such as a pneumothorax
- Smoker or living with a smoker
- Usual medication, particularly noting whether this includes steroids or theophylline
- Medication taken since attack started and its effectiveness

Key observations and findings
- Pulse: rate >110bpm
- Respiratory rate: tachypnoea >25bpm
- O_2 saturation should be monitored
- BP should be recorded at least every 30min
- Continuous cardiac monitoring
- Temperature: pyrexia suggest an infective cause

Key investigations
- PEFR: should be recorded if the patient is able. If the patient is unable to perform a PEFR urgent medical review is required
- Laboratory investigations: ABGs

Key actions and treatment
- Calm approach, as any sign of staff becoming excitable will exacerbate the feeling of rising panic already being experienced by the patient
- Immediate senior medical assessment
- 15L/min O_2 on non-rebreathing bag
- Drug therapy
  - 5mg salbutamol nebulized on O_2. Repeat PEFR 15–30min after nebulizer
  - IV hydrocortisone 200mg
  - If no improvement within 15min:
    —repeat salbutamol nebulizer
    —oral prednisolone 40mg
- After 60min if the PEFR is still <75% predicted or best the patient will require admission
- If the patient's condition deteriorates at any point urgent medical review is required and they should be treated as having life-threatening asthma

ⓘ **Moderate asthma**

Key signs and symptoms
- PEFR: 50–75% predicted or best
- Able to talk in short sentences

Key history and assessment
- Known asthmatic
- Previous admission for asthma
- Repeated use of inhaler without effect
- Exposure to known stimuli
- Chest pain: suggesting a complication such as a pneumothorax
- Smoker or living with a smoker
- Usual medication, particularly noting whether this includes steroids or theophylline
- Duration of symptoms, particularly wheeze, breathlessness, and nocturnal cough

Key observations and findings
- PEFR: 50–75% predicted or best value
- Pulse: rate normal or may be raised—particularly if the patient is deteriorating
- Respirations: rate normal or may be raised—particularly if the patient is deteriorating
- O₂ saturation should be monitored
- BP: should be recorded every 30min
- Temperature: pyrexia suggests infective cause, otherwise will be normal

Key investigations
- PEFR: 50–75% predicted value or best
- Laboratory investigations: ABGs

Key actions and treatment
- Calm approach so as not to exacerbate any feeling of rising panic already being experienced by the patient
- Early medical assessment
- Nebulizers: start with 5mg salbutamol
- Repeat PEFR 15–30min after nebulizer
- If PEFR still 50–75% repeat nebulizer
- Oral prednisolone 40mg
- Repeat PEFR after a further 30min:
  - PEFR <50%—treat as life threatening and obtain urgent medical review
  - PEFR 50–75%—repeat salbutamol and refer for admission
  - PEFR >75 %—continue to monitor
- After a further 60min repeat PEFR:
  - PEFR >75%—consider discharge
  - PEFR <75%—obtain urgent medical review

- On discharge the patient should be given oral and inhaled steroids, instructed to use their usual inhaled bronchodilator and be asked to make an early appointment with their Primary Care Service
- Instruct patient that if their condition worsens again before follow-up in primary care they must return to emergency care
- Encourage patient to present as early as possible in the event of a future asthma attack

⑦ Mild asthma

Key signs and symptoms
- PEFR: >75% predicted value or best
- Able to talk normally

Key history and assessment
- Known asthmatic
- Repeated use of inhaler without effect
- Smoker or living with a smoker
- Exposure to known stimuli
- Duration of symptoms: particularly wheeze, breathlessness and nocturnal cough
- Usual medication
- Events surrounding beginning of attack, to exclude possibility of hyperventilation
- Family history of atopic problems

Key observations and findings
- PEFR: >75% predicted value
- Pulse: rate normal
- Respirations: rate normal
- O_2 saturation
- BP: normal
- Temperature: pyrexia indicates infective cause, otherwise will be normal

Key investigations
- None normally required

Key actions and treatment
- Calm approach so as not to exacerbate any feeling of rising panic already being experienced by the patient
- Use patient's usual inhaled bronchodilator—take the opportunity to check their inhaler technique
- Repeat PEFR 30min after inhaler
- Medical assessment at this point
- PEFR: >75% at 60min—consider discharge
- On discharge the patient should be instructed to use their usual inhaled bronchodilator and be asked to make an early appointment with their Primary Care Service
- Instruct patient that if their condition worsens again before follow-up in primary care they must return to emergency care
- Encourage patient to present as early as possible in the event of a future asthma attack

Back pain

Differential diagnosis

☼ True emergencies
- Aortic aneurysm
- Cauda equina
- Spinal cord injury

☼ Urgent presentations
- Abdominal pathology
- Direct trauma to back

① Timely assessment
- Bony metastases
- Mechanical back pain
- Pathological fracture
- Pregnancy
- Prolapsed intervertebral disc

② Non-urgent presentations
- Arthritis
- Paget's disease.
- Shingles (herpes zoster)

Introduction

Back pain is a common presentation with >50% of the population experiencing it at some time. It occurs most often between the ages of 35–55 years. If the history is unclear and not related to direct trauma or mechanical injury then other pathology should be considered before the diagnosis of mechanical back pain is made.

Suspect underlying pathology if:
- Patient is <16 or >55 years old
- There is recent onset of pain without a history of trauma or lifting
- There is severe pain at rest
- There is bilateral sciatica
- There are urinary symptoms
- Vital signs are abnormal

There are many causes for back pain so it is important to establish a clear history and undertake a thorough examination in all cases.

History

The mnemonic PQRST can be used for describing the pain:
- **P:** Palliative/Provocative, what makes the pain better or worse?
- **Q:** Quality, sharp, dull, stabbing, burning, crushing, ache, nagging etc.
- **R:** Region/Radiation, where is the pain, where does it radiate to, especially to legs below knee level?
- **S:** Severity, record using pain scale
- **T:** Timing, when did the pain start, is it related to any event, is it worse first thing in the morning or late in the day?

Previous medical history
- Previous history of back problems
- What diagnosis was made and treatment suggested
- Osteoporosis
- Malignancies

Drug history
- Analgesia used and effect
- Steroid use

Occupation

Hobbies/sports played

Ability to pass urine and defaecate without incontinence

Any systemic symptoms

Examination
- Range of movement in spine with the patient erect and supine if possible
- Straight leg raising
- Muscle weakness
- Reflex loss
- Any numbness/tingling of legs or peri-anal area

☠ Aortic aneurysm

Lower back pain is a common feature of a leaking aortic aneurysm. This is a life threatening emergency and requires immediate medical attention.

📖 See Abdominal pain, p.1.

☠ Cauda equina syndrome

The spinal cord ends at the level of L1/L2 in most people. The bundle of nerve roots below this is known as the cauda equina and innervates the lower limbs and pelvic organs. Compression of these nerves will result in loss of sensation and function to the areas supplied, including bladder and anus. If not identified and treated early cauda equina compression can lead to permanent disability including loss of bowel and bladder control, loss of sexual function, and lower limb weakness.

Causes

Penetrating trauma
- Gunshot or stab wounds

Blunt trauma
- Blow to lower back
- Transmitted forces

Prolapsed intervertebral disc
- L4/L5 or L5/S1 are the commonest areas to be affected

Tumour
- Primary tumour
- Metastases

Infection
- Spinal abscess

Inflammation
- Exacerbation of existing inflammatory condition such as:
  - ankylosing spondylitis
  - paget's disease

Iatrogenic
- Following spinal surgery
- Spinal anaesthesia
- Lumbar puncture

Key signs and symptoms
- Lower back pain
- Altered or loss of sensation:
  - inner thighs and perineum—this is known as saddle anaesthesia
  - over the buttocks
  - back of legs
  - feet/heels
- Bladder and/or bowel dysfunction

Key history and assessment
- History of trauma
- Pre-existing causative factors

Key observations and findings
- Vital signs within normal parameters unless raised due to pain
- Reduced anal tone

- Diminished reflexes
- Reduced lower limb tone and strength

Key investigations

- XRs are of limited value
- CT/MRI
- Investigations should not delay the referral to the orthopaedic team
- FBC, U&E may be taken prior to surgery, but should not delay transfer to theatre

Key actions and treatment

- Analgesia
- Nil orally
- Urgent referral to the orthopaedic team
- Psychological support for the patient and their family
- Prevent potential injury to lower limbs which may have reduced sensation
- Pressure relieving aids may need to be used

☠ Spinal cord injury

Major or multiple trauma is the most common cause of spinal cord injury with the cervical section of the spine the area most often injured. The risk of an unstable spinal injury must be considered and managed with a spinal board or stable surface (such as a patient trolley), head blocks, tape and a semi rigid cervical collar, until cord injury has been excluded. Spinal immobilization can be very frightening for the patient, therefore clear explanations must be given at every stage of their care and treatment. Staff should ensure they stand within the visual field of the patient to enable eye contact to be made while talking, without the patient having to move their head or neck. Bony injury to the vertebrae can occur without spinal cord damage.

Spinal cord damage can occur in the absence of trauma as a result of infection, a cyst, or a tumour.

📖 See Neck pain, p.305.

☀ Abdominal pathology

Acute abdominal conditions such as pancreatitis, peptic ulcer and renal colic may present with back pain. These should be excluded before a diagnosis of mechanical back pain is made.

📖 see Abdominal pain, p.1.

✸ Direct trauma to back

Any patient reporting direct trauma to the back either with or without neurological signs and symptoms must be immobilized until assessed by an experienced practitioner.

Key signs and symptoms
- Pain:
  - assess using PQRST mnemonic
  - ask patient to point to exact location of the pain
- Reduced range of movement

Key history and assessment
- Direct blow to back, probably with a blunt object
- Fall onto protruding object
- Swelling
- Bruising
- Bony tenderness
- Abnormal steps on palpation of spinal column
- Anal tone
- Consider the possibility of other significant injuries

Key observations and findings
- Pulse: normal to slightly tachycardic due to pain or blood loss
- Respiratory rate: may be tachypnoeic depending on pain or blood loss
- O₂ saturation: should be normal unless associated chest injury is present
- BP: likely to be normal, unless significant blood loss has occurred

Key investigations
- Urinalysis
- Pregnancy test in women of childbearing age
- Spinal XR

Key actions and treatment
- Analgesia:
  - paracetamol 1g either orally or IV
  - codeine 60mg
  - NSAIDs
  - IV opiates if pain severe
- Diazepam 5mg orally to relax muscles
- Monitor abnormal sensation and ability to urinate/defaecate
- Refer to orthopaedics if bony injury present or pain not resolving
- Consider referral to spinal unit if unstable fracture or any neurological signs
- If no bony injury and pain managed successfully then attempt mobilization

① **Bony metastases**

A number of primary tumours can metastasize to the spinal column. The most common are breast, prostate, lung, and renal. The patient presenting as an emergency normally does so as a result of pain. They may or may not be aware of a primary diagnosis.

Key signs and symptoms
- Pain:
  - use PQRST mnemonic
  - ask patient to point to exact location of the pain
- Reduced range of movement due to pain

Key history and assessment
- Previous or current malignancy
- Abnormal neurological signs

Key observations and findings
- Pulse: normal to slightly tachycardic due to pain or pre-existing condition
- Respiratory rate: may be tachypnoeic depending on degree of pain and level of injury
- O₂ saturation: should be normal
- BP: likely to be normal, depending on any pre-existing condition

Key investigations
- Urinalysis
- Spinal XRs: any pain without trauma is suspicious

Key actions and treatment
- Analgesia:
  - paracetamol 1g orally or IV
  - codeine 60mg
  - NSAIDs.
  - IV opiates if pain severe
- Monitor abnormal sensation and ability to urinate/defaecate
- Refer for admission

① Mechanical back pain

The vast majority of back pain presentations will be due to simple mechanical pain as a result of ligamentous or muscular injury. Causes include:
- Poor posture
- Repetitive twisting and bending:
  - production-line work
  - moving furniture
  - carrying shopping
  - gardening
- Stretching up to high shelves
- Sport

Sometimes there is a relatively low level trigger, which is sufficient to cause severe pain on top of underlying back problems. The adoption of good manual handling practices should be encouraged wherever possible, especially with healthcare workers.

Key signs and symptoms
- Pain:
  - use PQRST mnemonic
  - ask patient to point to exact location of pain
- Able to walk but may have difficulty
- Restricted range of movement in spine

Key history and assessment
- Poor manual handling practice
- Pain exacerbated on movement
- No bony tenderness
- No signs of infection
- Check straight leg raising
- Ensure no muscle weakness
- Ensure reflexes are present and normal
- Check anal tone
- Check for any loss of sensation

Key observations and findings
- All observations are usually normal

Key investigations
- None in otherwise healthy young patients
- XRs may be considered in order to exclude osteoporosis or other conditions

Key actions and treatment
- Analgesia:
  - paracetamol 1g
  - codeine 60mg
  - NSAIDs
- Diazepam 5mg to relax muscles
- Encourage to mobilize 1 hour after analgesia, by when pain relief should be adequate

- Back care advice prior to discharge. This should include:
  - correct manual handling practice
  - use of ice packs for the first 48 hours
  - use of warm packs after the first 48 hours
  - mobilizing gently within limits of pain
  - regular analgesia and written instructions on how to use it
  - patients should not be advised to try bed rest as this increases muscle stiffness and pain
- The patient should be advised to arrange follow up in primary care if the condition is not improving after 2–3 days

⚠ Pathological fracture

A pathological fracture may occur when the bone is weakened by a concurrent disease process such as tumor, cyst, infection, or an inherited bone disorder. Treatment needs to be focused on both the management of the fracture and the underlying problem.

Key signs and symptoms
- Pain:
  - use PQRST mnemonic
  - ask patient to point to exact location of pain
- Reduced range of movement

Key history and assessment
- Post-menopausal
- Prolonged steroid use
- Known osteoporosis
- Known malignancy
- Severity of pain out of proportion to mechanism of injury
- Weight loss
- Systemically unwell

Key observations and findings
- Vital signs will vary depending on the underlying pathological process
- Pulse, BP, respiratory rate and temperature should be recorded

Key investigations
- Urinalysis
- Spinal XR: any pain with little or no trauma is suspicious

Key actions and treatment
- Analgesia:
  - paracetamol 1g
  - codeine 60mg
  - NSAIDs
- Diazepam 5mg to relax muscles
- Keep patient immobile until XR results available
- Monitor abnormal sensation and ability to urinate/defaecate
- Refer to orthopaedics if pathology discovered
- If osteoporosis diagnosed refer to primary care for further investigation and treatment

① **Pregnancy**

Up to 75% of pregnant women experience back pain with a minority also developing sciatica.

Two different types of back pain occur. The first is similar to simple mechanical back pain whereby the ligaments, muscles, and intervertebral discs are put under pressure as a result of altered posture. Pain often increases during the day and can be relieved by rest, application of gentle heat, exercise, and avoiding heavy lifting.

The other type, pelvic girdle pain, is more common. During pregnancy the ligaments in the pelvis start to relax in preparation for delivery. This enables the normally stable pelvic joints to move slightly and places stress on the pelvic structures which results in pain and inflammation. Pelvic girdle pain is normally unilateral and may be felt in the buttocks with shooting pains down the back of the legs. This often leads to it being mis-diagnosed as sciatica, but sensory disturbance is absent. It may also alternate from one side to the other and is worse at night when lying down.

Conventional management may exacerbate peluic girdle pain. The most effective form of treatment is exercise to stabilize the abdominal and pelvic floor muscles, in combination with the use of a pelvic support belt. Teaching patients how to stabilize the pelvis whilst undertaking activities can be helpful. Early referral to a community midwife or the obstetric team for further support may be useful.

① Prolapsed intervertebral disc

Prolapse of an intervertebral disc may put pressure on the nerve root. The condition commonly affects L3, L4, L5, and S1. The resulting pain is known as sciatica, as the sciatic nerve roots are often affected.

Key signs and symptoms
- Pain:
  - use PQRST mnemonic
  - severe
  - unilateral
  - pain deep in the buttock
  - radiating down the inner aspect of the thigh
  - may extend down to the foot
- Able to walk, but may be dragging one foot or limping due to sciatic nerve injury

Key history and assessment
- Pain may be worse on forward flexion, coughing, or sneezing
- Saddle anaesthesia
- Sudden onset of incontinence due to loss of sphincter control

Key observations and findings
- Vital signs are usually normal
- Pulse, BP, respiratory rate and temperature should be recorded

Key investigations
- Urinalysis
- Spinal XR: to exclude bony injury or other pathology
- Any pain with little or no trauma is suspicious

Key actions and treatment
- Analgesia:
  - paracetamol 1g
  - codeine 60mg
  - NSAIDs
- Diazepam 5mg to relax muscles
- Monitor abnormal sensation and ability to urinate/defaecate
- Refer to orthopaedics if neurological abnormalities are present

⑦ Arthritis/Paget's disease

Most patients with arthritis or Paget's disease will already have a diagnosis and should not present as an emergency with back pain. It is possible they may present if in more pain than usual or they have run out of analgesia, particularly if away from home. Provided they report no new symptoms they should be treated with oral analgesia and referred back to primary care for further management.

⑦ Shingles (herpes zoster)

Reactivation of a latent infection along a peripheral sensory nerve tract by the varicella zoster virus. It is more common in the elderly and depending on the nerve involved may present with unilateral back pain.

📖 See Rashes, p.353.

Behaving strangely

Differential diagnosis

☻ True emergencies
- Aggression
- Alcohol withdrawal syndrome
- Diabetic ketoacidosis
- Hypoglycaemia
- Raised intracranial pressure

☼ Urgent presentations
- Alcohol
- Dehydration
- Substance misuse

① Timely assessment
- Constipation
- Electrolyte imbalance
- Head injury
- Post-ictal

Introduction

There is a tendency to put 'strange behaviour' down to mental illness. This should be resisted unless organic causes for the behaviour have been investigated and eliminated. Only then should a mental health assessment be made to determine the level of risk the patient poses to themselves and others. The causes discussed in the rest of this chapter of 'strange' or 'abnormal' behaviour need to be ruled out.

☠ Aggression

Aggression may be either physical or verbal. The majority of aggressive and violent incidents are not perpetrated by people with mental health problems, but more often than not occur as a result of alcohol intoxication, substance misuse, or confusional states. A duty of care exists to colleagues and other patients, as well as to the aggressive person. Staff need to balance these, often conflicting, duties and should not hesitate to call for security staff or police should the situation warrant it.

Conditions associated with aggressive behaviour

- Alcohol intoxication or withdrawal
- Electrolyte imbalance
- Hypoxia
- Hypoglycaemia
- Encephalitis
- Meningitis
- Traumatic head injury
- Intracerebral bleed
- Subarachnoid bleed
- Subdural haematoma
- Personality disorder
- Psychosis
- Substance intoxication or withdrawal
- Post-traumatic stress disorder

Most aggressive incidents are preceded by a number of warning signs and staff need to be able to recognize these and act to defuse situations to prevent violence occurring if at all possible.

Key signs and symptoms

- Non verbal:
  - tense or agitated appearance
  - entering personal space
  - increased activity, restless, inability to stay still—agitation
  - balling of fist
  - unusual or inconsistent behaviour
  - abusive gestures
  - rapid breathing
  - sweating
  - dilated pupils

- Verbal:
  - abrupt conversation style
  - raised voice
  - obscenities
  - abusive comments

Key history and assessment

- Known history of violence
- Violence threatened
- Alcohol intoxication
- Substance misuse
- Head injury
- Post-seizure
- Mental health problems
- Personality disorder
- Unrealistic expectations of service or treatment
- Stress
- Frustration
- Feelings of inadequacy
- Anxiety
- Fear
- Perceived unsympathetic attitude from staff
- Perceived discrimination

Key observations and findings

It may be necessary to eliminate an organic cause if possible and safe to do so:

- Pulse: tachycardia
- Respiratory rate: tachypnoeic—hypoxia
- Capillary blood glucose—hypoglycemia

Key actions and treatment

Verbal aggression

- Consider requesting the presence of security staff (if available) prior to seeing patient
- Communicate at a safe distance: stay at least one arm's length away from the patient
- Maintain an exit route at all times:
  - keep a door open
  - ensure the patient does not come between you and the door
  - inform colleagues of the situation
- If possible, attempt to defuse the situation:
  - calm, confident manner
  - objective, non-critical approach
  - take time to listen and talk
  - demonstrate concern and understanding
  - acknowledge the feelings and emotions of the person
  - try to clarify the patient's concerns
  - do not over-react to the patient's emotions
  - do not get drawn into an argument

- Use non threatening body language
- If you are unable to defuse the situation withdraw and let someone else speak to the patient or request security support if appropriate
- Physical restraint should be used if there is a risk of harm occurring and then only as a last resort by staff trained in restraint techniques
- Sedation may be considered if the patient's agitated state poses a danger to themselves or others. Local guidelines should be followed

Physical assault

- If a physical assault is threatened your priority should be to escape from the situation as quickly as possible
- Call for help
- Use panic button to notify security if available
- If the attacker has a weapon of any kind, withdraw at once and call the Police

All aggressive, threatening or violent behaviour should be reported to the Police.

Consider speaking to a clinical supervisor, Occupational Health service, or psychological support worker in order to minimize the potential effects on yourself.

☣ Alcohol withdrawal syndrome

Acute withdrawal from alcohol consumption can occur in anyone who is a regular heavy drinker. Alcohol withdrawal causes a wide range of symptoms and signs which usually occur within 6–12 hours of cessation. In 1–5% of people withdrawing from alcohol dependency delirium tremens, commonly known as the DTs, may develop. This is a life-threatening condition with mortality of 5–35%. As such it should be treated as a medical emergency. Patients may not have the mental capacity to consent to treatment and may have to be treated initially 'in their best interest'. DTs do not occur until 24–72 hours after withdrawal and may last up to 10 days, commonly peaking at 7 days.

Alcohol withdrawal may occur whilst the patient has alcohol on board; a sudden reduction in the quantity of alcohol consumed may be sufficient to cause symptoms therefore, do *not* assume that a patient is not in withdrawal if alcohol is present.

Key signs and symptoms

- Alcohol withdrawal syndrome:
  - sweating
  - N&V
  - anxiety, agitation
  - skin flushes
  - hand tremor
  - upper abdominal pain
  - convulsions
- DTs:
  - acute confusional state
  - paranoia
  - disorientation
  - profuse sweating
  - cardiovascular collapse may occur
  - autonomic overactivity—tachycardia, high BP, dilated pupils, etc.
  - hallucinations, visual and tactile may occur, often inanimate objects such as patterns on curtains are seen to be moving. Also spiders or rats seen climbing walls or felt as insects or spiders crawling on the skin

Key history and assessment

- History of previous alcohol intake—quantity and any recent reduction in intake
- Pre-existing medical conditions
- Depression
- Insomnia
- Impulsive behaviour
- Disinhibition
- Impaired concentration
- Short-term memory loss
- Contact with police

Key observations and findings
- Pulse: tachycardia
- Temperature: pyrexia
- Respiratory rate: tachypnoea
- BP: hypertension

Key investigations
- Blood glucose
- FBC, U&Es, LFTs

Key actions and treatment
- Refer to medical team for management of physical signs and symptoms
- Admit to HDU if necessary—patients with DT
- Mild withdrawal may require no intervention other than support and observation
- If required IV access and IV fluids
- Benzodiazepines can help with anxiety and agitation, and they reduce the likelihood of withdrawal seizures
- IV thiamine
- Haloperidol for agitation and hallucinations if required

☠ Diabetic ketoacidosis

Diabetic ketoacidosis (which may occur either in new onset or poorly controlled diabetes) may present with confusion or aggression. Ketones will be found in the urine along with high blood glucose levels.

📖 See Diabetes, p.157.

☠ Hypoglycaemia

Very low blood glucose may cause confusion and aggression.

📖 See Diabetes, p.157.

☠ Raised intracranial pressure

Swelling of the brain or an increase in the volume of cerebrospinal fluid (CSF) may cause the pressure within the skull to rise. This may compress the blood vessels resulting in poor cerebral perfusion. This will result in a deterioration of the patient's conscious level. Signs of this include increasing restlessness, purposeless activity, and confusion.

📖 See Headache, p.251, and Head injury, p.269.

☼ Alcohol

Alcohol affects the behaviour of different people in different ways. The effect depends on the amount consumed, the age and gender of the person and any alcohol tolerance he/she may have developed.

The effects of alcohol include:
- Loss of social inhibition
- Poor coordination
- Slurred speech
- Aggression
- Violence
- Drowsiness

The definitive way of establishing whether alcohol is making any contribution to the patient's behaviour is to measure breath alcohol content with an alcometer. A positive breath test does **not** exclude other causes of strange behaviour. A negative result excludes alcohol as the cause of the patient's condition.

Do not dismiss any patient as 'just drunk'. A patient with a reduced level of consciousness may have airway problems regardless of the cause. Be aware that alcohol absorption can continue for up to 2 hours following the last drink. The patient who appears to be calming down may be experiencing a lowering of his/her conscious level. Regular neuro observations are extremely important in this group.

Patients in whom alcohol has been identified as the cause of their behaviour should only be discharged when they are able to protect their airway and if accompanied by a responsible adult who will stay with them until they are sober.

📖 See Apparently drunk, p.37.

:☼: Dehydration

Patients become dehydrated for a variety of reasons. These include: diarrhoea and vomiting, infection, inadequate fluid intake, and polyuria (diabetes, diuretics etc.).

Key signs and symptoms
- Dry skin
- Thirst
- Oliguria: normal response to dehydration
- Polyuria: abnormal response, consider diabetes or diuretics
- Dizziness
- Drowsiness: if dehydration is severe
- Confusion: if dehydration is severe

Key history and assessment
- History of clinical deterioration
- Increasing drowsiness and confusion
- Aggression
- Thorough questioning may be needed to elicit exact food and fluid intake and urine output
- History of diarrhoea and vomiting
- History of infection
- Extended period of physical activity (such as endurance events) with inadequate fluid intake
- Periods of unusually hot weather

Key observations and findings
- Reduced skin turgor in young patients
- Dry tongue
- Sunken eyes
- Pulse: tachycardia is common
- Respiratory rate:
  - tachypnoea
  - O_2 saturation <94%—may be difficult to record
- BP: hypotension is a late sign and indicates severe dehydration
- Temperature: may be raised due to underlying infection

Key investigations
- Laboratory investigations:
  - FBC: baseline
  - U&E: baseline for renal function—a raised urea is consistent with dehydration
  - Blood glucose

Key actions and treatment
- Medical assessment
- Encourage oral fluids
- High-dose O_2 via a non-rebreathing mask, unless history of chronic obstructive pulmonary disease
- Hourly neuro observations
- IV access should be considered if unable to tolerate oral fluids
- Consider admission

☼ Substance misuse

People abuse a vast range of drugs and other substances for a variety of reasons. Some will abuse more than one substance at the same time.

📖 See Overdose and poisoning, p.313, and Self-harm, p.361

Key signs and symptoms
- Needle tracks on:
  - forearms
  - groins
  - between digits
  - base of penis in men
- Abscesses over old needle tracks, in axillae and in groins
- Signs of damage to nose, particularly septum: suggestive of cocaine use
- Wet or acne-type 'spots' around nose and mouth: suggestive of solvent abuse
- Limited attention span
- Agitation
- Cold sweats, shivering: suggestive of withdrawal

May also present with:
- Visual hallucinations
- Auditory hallucinations
- Paranoia
- Aggression
- Violence

Key history and assessment
- Be objective rather than judgemental
- Obtain clear history of the nature of substances involved
- Amount taken and frequency of use.
- Ask specifically about the possibility of deliberate overdose

Key observations and findings
- Pulse and BP:
  - may be tachycardic depending on substance taken
  - BP may be abnormal depending on substance taken
- Capillary blood glucose: check for hyperglycaemia and hypoglycaemia
- Cardiac monitoring may be necessary if the pulse or BP are abnormal
- Respiratory rate:
  - likely to be normal
  - respiratory depression may be found in opiate overdose
  - tachypnoea may be found in amphetamine overdose
- Temperature: ecstasy (MDMA) use can cause hyperpyrexia and severe dehydration.

Key investigations
- 12-lead ECG: in all patients with new confusion or tachycardia.
- Laboratory studies:
  - baseline FBC, U&Es

- paracetamol and salicylate levels are useful if deliberate overdose is considered
- toxicology screens are rarely helpful in the initial phase of treatment, unless an unknown toxin is suspected. If the police want a toxicology screen it must be taken by a police surgeon, with the patient's consent and processed by the forensic service

Key actions and treatment
- Dependent on severity of symptoms
- May need admission for treatment of toxicity
- May need psychiatry assessment once signs of toxicity have resolved
- Consider referral to local substance misuse service

! Constipation

Constipation can be a cause of abnormal behaviour in the elderly, very young, or those with learning disabilities.

  📖 See Abdominal pain, p.1.

! Electrolyte imbalance

If electrolyte levels (particularly sodium and potassium) are abnormal the patient's behaviour can be significantly affected.

Key signs and symptoms
- Confusion
- Agitation
- Collapse

Key history and assessment
- Elderly and very young children are particularly vulnerable
- History of diarrhoea and/or vomiting
- New drug treatment: particularly diuretics
- Reluctance to eat and drink-check possibility of swallowing problems

Key observations and findings
- Pulse: may be abnormal if hypo/hyperkalaemia is present
- Respiratory rate: usually normal
- BP: usually normal but may be low if arrhythmias occur
- Temperature: may be raised in systemic infection
- O_2 saturation: monitoring is required
- Capillary blood glucose should always be recorded
- Cardiac monitoring is required if any electrolyte imbalance is suspected

Key investigations
- Laboratory studies:
  - FBC: likely to be normal
  - U&E: pay particular attention to sodium and potassium levels
  - blood glucose
- 12-lead ECG

Key actions and treatment
- Observations at least every 30min
- IV access
- Fluid prescription to address deficits over 24–48-hour period
- Experienced medical advice is required if any electrolyte abnormalities are present
- Admission under the care of the physicians

⚠ Head injury

Head injured patients often present in a confused, disorientated state.

📖 See Head injury, p.269.

⚠ Post-ictal

Patients who have had an epileptic fit can present with confusion and disorientation.

📖 See Fits, p.225.

Bites and stings

Differential diagnosis

☼ True emergencies
- Anaphylaxis
- Bites causing major structural damage
- Tetanus

① Timely assessment
- Animal and human bites
- Infection
- Specific treatments

② Non urgent presentation
- Local reactions

Introduction

Most people will suffer a bite or a sting at some time. For the vast majority this results in a minor wound or local irritation. For some it may cause permanent damage or incapacity and a few will face a life- or limb-threatening emergency as a result of major haemorrhage, massive tissue loss, over-whelming infection, or anaphylaxis. Bites are caused by humans, animals, or insects, with dog bites accounting for up to 90% of all incidents. Stings are usually caused by insects, plants, or marine animals. Treatment is easier if the causative agent is known. Beyond the initial pain and haemorrhage which may accompany a bite or sting the most common problem is that of wound infection, which must be managed appropriately in order to prevent the development of cellulitis, osteomyelitis, or septicaemia.

☠️ Anaphylaxis

A severe reaction, sometimes fatal, occurring upon exposure to a foreign material such as a wasp or bee sting. The patient rapidly becomes systemically unwell. Patients with a history of previous anaphylaxis or those thought to be at high risk may carry an auto injector of epinephrine (adrenaline), such as an EpiPen® or Anapen® which can be self-administered at the onset of an attack.

📖 See Allergy, p.31.

☠️ Bites causing major structural damage

Treatment will depend on presentation, which will vary. Large mammals such as dogs can cause life- and limb-threatening injuries, and in some areas large marine animals can also inflict serious damage. These should be treated as major trauma.

📖 See Major trauma, p.293.

☠️ Tetanus

An acute disease of the nervous system, caused by the contamination of wounds by *Clostridium tetani* which can be found in animal faeces and soil. It may be transmitted via animal bites (especially deep puncture wounds) and soil contamination of open wounds.

📖 See Wounds, p.427.

ⓘ Animal and human bites

All animal and human bites are potentially infected; however, the balance of evidence suggests that dog bites should not routinely be given prophylactic antibiotics, whereas human and cat bites should. This should be confirmed by local policy. Human bites are particularly likely to become infected. Bites from large dogs may cause underlying bone injury. The sharp needle-like teeth of cats may damage tendon sheaths. Rabies should be considered if the bite occurred in a rabies risk zone.

Key signs and symptoms
- Obvious wound
- Presence of infection

Key history and assessment
- Mechanism of injury
- Time of injury
- Place of injury
- Pain
- Fever
- Allergies
- Tetanus immunization history
- Consider potential for rabies infection—in affected regions

Key observations and findings
- Size of wound
- Depth of wound
- Shape of wound
- Location of wound
- Involvement of structures underlying the skin
- Ability to move affected part normally
- Sensory abnormalities

Key investigations
- Establish accurate tetanus immunization history from GP or relatives, if necessary
- Ensure no tooth fragments remain in the wound as a FB. May require XR

Key actions and treatment
- Thorough cleaning of wound: tap water first, followed by irrigation with normal saline
- Careful examination of wound to establish degree of damage
- Refer for further assessment and repair if any bone or tendon damage is found or major reconstruction is required. Local policy will differ as to which specialty manages these injuries
- In general, wounds should not be closed. Leaving them open will reduce the risk of abscess formation. If the wound must be closed, use adhesive strips with gaps in between as this allows discharge to escape. Sutures or glue should be avoided. The exception to this rule is facial wounds which should be closed for cosmetic reasons
- If the injury is on the hand or forearm a high arm sling should be applied for 24 hours
- Advice on wound care should be given
- Local policy should be followed with regard to the use of antibiotics

① Infection

If a bite is >6 hours old when first seen it should be considered to be infected. Many patients presenting with infected bites or stings will have suffered the initial incident 2 or 3 days previously. Human and cat bites are the most likely to become infected. Beware of puncture wounds to the knuckles occurring as a result of striking someone in the mouth as this constitutes a human bite.

Key signs and symptoms
- One or more wounds
- Redness and warmth of skin
- Pain
- Swelling around wound
- Red 'tracking' along route of lymphatic system
- Sensory abnormalities, suggesting nerve injury
- Restricted range of movement
- Discharge or blistering

Key history and assessment
- Mechanism of injury
- Associated injuries
- Time and place of injury
- Pain
- Allergies
- Tetanus immunization history
- Signs of systemic infection
- Consider potential for rabies infection—in affected regions

Key observations and findings
- Vital signs usually normal unless sepsis present

Key investigations
- None normally required
- XR required if wound overlies a joint and/or possibility of a FB present

Key actions and treatment
- Thorough cleaning of wound with tap water
- Careful examination of wound and surrounding area to establish degree of damage
- Mark limits of redness and any tracking with indelible marker
- Consider closing wound—particularly face
- Antibiotics for all patients presenting with an established infection
- Follow-up needed, usually in primary care
- Admission for IV antibiotics for those with signs of systemic infection
- Keep infected part elevated if possible

⚠ Specific treatments

A number of specific animals merit individual consideration due to the prevalence of presentation or public concern.

Bee stings
- Bees often leave a sting in situ
- Scrape the sting out if possible
- Do not pull as this may inject further venom
- Wash with sodium bicarbonate solution
- Oral analgesia such as paracetamol 1g

Wasp stings
- Wash the area in vinegar to neutralize the irritation
- Oral analgesia such as paracetamol 1g

Snake bites

Snake bites are universally feared around the world, and although potentially fatal, in reality are rarely so. In the USA it is estimated that approximately 8000 people a year are bitten, with an annual death rate of around 5 people. In Australia a similar ratio is found with 3000 bites and 1 or 2 fatalities. <10% of all people bitten require treatment with anti-venom and the risks associated with this treatment are not to be taken lightly.

Key signs and symptoms
- The sequencing and time of onset of signs and symptoms can vary widely from a few minutes to several hours. This will depend the individual circumstances and is difficult to predict
- The bite itself may not be painful
- Bruising around the bite site, may obscure bite marks
- Bleeding
- Localized swelling
- Headache
- N&V
- Diarrhoea
- Confusion
- Irritability
- Photophobia
- Lymphadenopathy
- Further signs and symptoms are related to the neurotoxicty, coagulopathic, and myotoxic effects of the venom and all require specialist critical care

Key actions and treatment
- Most venom is spread via the lymphatic system and the aim of the initial treatment is to slow the rate of absorption and prevent the spread of the venom centrally
- Pad and firmly bandage directly over the bite site, even if not on a limb
- Continue the bandage as far towards the centre of the body as possible
- Splint the area if possible
- Immobilize the patient

- Do not remove any bandage until the patient is in a critical care environment
- Provide psychological support to the patient
- Manage any symptoms as appropriate
- Do not try to remove or suck out any venom
- Do not apply a tourniquet
- Obtain expert help if available

Weever fish

Weever fish inhabit the waters of the North Atlantic, the English Channel, and the Mediterranean, spending most of their time buried just under the surface of the sand. The greater weever can grow up to 50cm long but is most often found in deeper waters. More commonly it is the lesser weever fish, normally about 10cm long, that is stood on by unsuspecting bathers. The weever fish has between 5–7 spines on its dorsal fin which contain a neurotoxic venom that is injected into the sole of the victims foot.

Key signs and symptoms
- Localized:
  - severe pain at the site
  - intense itching
  - swelling around the site and in the affected part
  - heat
  - redness
  - numbness
  - tingling
- Joint ache
- Headache
- Abdominal cramp
- N&V
- Tremor
- Cardiac arrhythmias
- Generalized weakness
- Shortness of breath
- Hypotension
- Seizures
- Paralysis

Key history and assessment
- History of sudden, intense pain
- Paddling in shallow water
- Patient often think they have stood on glass

Key actions and treatment
- Use tweezers to remove any spines in the wound
- Do not touch with bare hands
- Immerse the affected area in water as hot as the person who has been stung can tolerate:
  - toxin breaks down in temperatures of around 40°C
  - be careful not to scald the patient. Placing a non-affected part in the hot water first helps to assess the temperature and minimize the risk of scalding

- Repeat as necessary to control pain
- Clean wound with soap and water
- Irrigate extensively with fresh water
- Oral analgesia
- Do not cover the wound

Jellyfish

Jellyfish are found throughout the world's seas and oceans and number several thousand species. Reports on which are, or are not, toxic to humans vary, with very little consensus. It would appear that some people can come into contact and suffer no ill effects, while others will find it a very painful experience. In general those species found in temperate waters are less likely to be harmful than those in tropical areas. The box jellyfish, found of the coast of Australia, is considered to be the most venomous creature on earth. To put the problem into perspective, it is thought that >50,000 jellyfish stings occur around the world each year and in Australia, a total of 63 deaths have been documented since record keeping began.

Key signs and symptoms

- Pain
- Burning sensation
- Redness
- Itching

Key history and assessment

- Contact with jellyfish while in the sea
- Sudden on set of symptoms while in the sea without known contact

Key actions and treatment

- Avoid contact with toxin
- Wash area with sea water—do not use fresh water as there are reports this can increase pain
- Vinegar may help to neutralize toxin. Large quantities will be required
- Ice or heat may help to ease pain
- Oral analgesia
- Observe for signs of infection over following days

⑦ Local reactions

Local reactions are more common in stings, particularly plants. They normally are the result of excessive histamine release in response to the irritant.

Key signs and symptoms
- Redness, possibly with hives
- Skin warm to touch
- Swelling
- Pain
- Itching

Key history and assessment
- Causative agent
- Associated injuries
- Time of injury
- Place of injury
- Pain
- Allergies
- Extent of reaction
- Location of reaction
- Appearance of reaction
- Ability to feel normal sensation
- Ability to move affected part normally

Key observations and findings
- Vital signs should all be normal

Key investigations
- None required

Key actions and treatment
- Discussion with patient on self-management of hives, itching and pain—these are likely to subside within 24 hours
- Consider the requirement for oral antihistamines and analgesia to provide comfort as reaction wears off
- Beware of the potential for airway involvement in anyone with reactions on their face
- Topical antihistamines are rarely effective and can increase the local irritation

Burns and scalds

Differential diagnosis

☀ True emergencies
- Major burns
- Inhalation injury

☼ Urgent presentations
- Chemical burns
- Circumferential burns
- Electrical burns
- Facial burns

① Timely assessment
- Hand burns
- Perineal burns
- Superficial burns

⑦ Non-urgent presentations
- Sunburn

Introduction

Burns and scalds can be defined as injuries caused by heat, electricity, irradiation, or chemicals. An understanding of the mechanism of injury is necessary to appreciate the nature and potential extent of the damage caused and therefore the risks to the patient. However, resuscitation measures must not be delayed while obtaining a history of the incident. Past medical history of cardiac or respiratory problems is important as it can affect the outcome for the patient.

Mechanism of injury

In determining the mechanism of injury it is important to ascertain:
- Exact time of the injury?
- What was the source of the injury?
- Nature of any materials involved?:
  - risk of inhalation burns
  - increased exposure to noxious fumes
  - carbon monoxide (CO) poisoning
- Was the fire in an enclosed space?
- Was there an explosion?:
  - associated blast injuries
  - head injury
  - injury to tympanic membranes
- Loss of consciousness?
- Length of exposure?

First aid

First aid is essential to minimize the extent of the injury:
- Safely remove patient from source of the burn whilst maintaining your own safety
- Assess the airway and maintain if required
- Stop the burning process by applying cold water to reduce heat in tissues
- Avoid causing hypothermia
- Remove any corrosive substance, *taking care not to contaminate yourself*
- Remove any constricting jewellery and any metal which may concentrate heat
- Do not remove burnt clothing which is adherent to the skin
- Protect damaged skin by covering it with something clean and light—cling film is ideal
- Give analgesia

Extent of burn

The depth and extent of the burn must be assessed (ignoring simple erythema). The extent of the burn is expressed as a percentage of the total body surface area (TBSA). If available, Lund and Browder charts are commonly used. (Fig. 10.1).

(a)

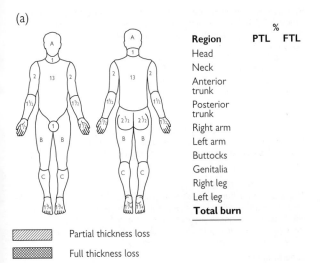

Region	PTL	% FTL
Head		
Neck		
Anterior trunk		
Posterior trunk		
Right arm		
Left arm		
Buttocks		
Genitalia		
Right leg		
Left leg		
Total burn		

▨▨▨ Partial thickness loss

▨▨▨ Full thickness loss

(b) Relative percentage of body surface area affected by growth

AREA	AGE 0	AGE 1	AGE 5	AGE 10	AGE 15	ADULT
A = ½ of head	9 ½	8 ½	6 ½	5 ½	4 ½	3 ½
B = ½ of one thigh	2 ¾	3 ¼	4	4 ½	4 ½	4 ¾
C = ½ of one leg	2 ½	2 ½	2 ¾	3	3 ¼	3 ½

Fig. 10.1 (a) and (b) Lund and Browder charts

Wallace's rule of nines (Fig. 10.2) can also be used to provide a rough estimate. With this method the body is divided up into areas which can be divided or multiplied by 9%, with the exception of the perineum which is assessed as 1%:

- Head, front, and back: 9%
- Arms, front, and back: 9%
- Chest and abdomen: 18%
- Back: 18%
- Legs, front, and back: 18%
- Perineum: 1%

It is also possible to roughly estimate the percentage using the patient's hand as a guide to 1% of their body surface area. If using this method, the whole hand from the base of the palm to the tips of the fingers constitutes the 1%

Depth of burn

The depth of the burn is classified as partial or full thickness. Partial thickness burns are subdivided in superficial or deep dermal. Superficial burns which consist of simple erythema *are not included* in the assessment of the extent of the injury. In some areas of the world, the classification of 1st-, 2nd-, and 3rd-degree burns is still used.

Superficial burns:
- Epidermis only
- Erythema
- Mild discomfort
- Heals within 3–4 days without intervention
- No scarring
- Not counted in burn assessment

Superficial partial thickness:
- Effects the epidermis and upper layers of the dermis
- Moist
- Painful
- Hypersensitivity
- Heals within 2–3 weeks
- Minimal scarring

Deep partial thickness:
- Extends to the subcutaneous (SC) tissue
- White and mottled skin
- Area is non-blanching
- Painful
- 4 weeks to heal
- Grafting is normally required

Full thickness:
- Epidermis and dermis destroyed
- Muscle, fat, tendon, and bone may be involved
- Skin white or brown, dry, and leathery
- No capillary refill
- Painless with absent sensation
- Grafting is required

In most patients with significant burns a combination of burn depths will be present and it is not always easy to ascertain accurately at first the exact extent of the burn and its depth.

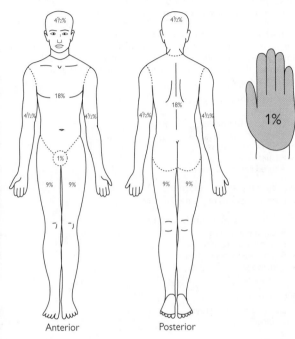

Fig. 10.2 Wallace's rule of nines

☠ Major burns

In an adult any burn >15% TBSA will require fluid resuscitation and is therefore classified as a major burn. Full thickness burns of 5% TBSA are also classed as major, along with those which affect the airway or affect particular areas of the body such as the hands, eyes, or perineum. As soon as the injury occurs the capillaries start leaking plasma. This can continue for up to 36 hours and leads to tissue oedema. As a result of the fluid loss, hypovolaemia and haemoconcentration may occur. This leads to poor perfusion; if this situation is allowed to continue the patient quickly becomes shocked.

Key signs and symptoms
- Skin pallor
- Cold and clammy skin
- Thirst and cold
- Respiratory distress
- Restlessness
- Altered conscious level

Key history and assessment
- Burn area of 15% or greater in adults

Key observations and findings
- Rapid, thready pulse
- Poor capillary refill
- Rapid, shallow respirations
- Reduced urinary output
- Tissue oedema

Key investigations
- Laboratory investigations
  - blood gases
  - U&E
  - FBC
  - carboxyhaemoglobin
  - group and save
- 12-lead ECG
- CXR if respiratory involvement suspected

Key actions and treatment
- Assess airway, breathing, and circulation
- Give 100% humidified O_2
- Insert 2 large-bore cannulae
- IV fluid resuscitation will be required in accordance with local guidelines
- Cardiac monitor
- Pulse oximetry
- Regular observations
- Analgesia
- Tetanus prophylaxis if required
- Urinary catheter

- Monitor fluid balance with hourly urine measurement
- Cover or dress burns with cling film
- Admit to burns unit or ICU as appropriate
- Provide support for relatives

Fluid replacement

If the TBSA exceeds 10% the patient will require IV fluid resuscitation. The most appropriate fluid to use is still the subject of debate and local guideline should be followed.

A number of different formulas are available for calculating the quantity of fluid required. The Parkland formula and the Muir and Barclay formula being the two most widely used. Adherence to local practice should be followed.

Parkland formula

This formula is based on the use of crystalloid solution (such as Hartmann's solution) for the first 24 hours *following the incident* (not arrival at the health care facility) and uses 4 mL × patient's weight in kg × percentage area of burn.

Example

For an 80kg patient with 20% TBSA burns using the lower figure:

$$4mL \times 80 \text{ kg} \times 20\% = 6400mL$$

- 50% of this quantity is given in the first 8 hours post-injury
- 50% given in the next 16 hours

Muir and Barclay formula

This formula divides the immediate 36 hours post-injury into three 12-hour blocks during which a set amount of colloid is administered. The quantity of fluid required in each time period first needs to be determined using the following calculation:

$$\frac{\text{Percentage area of burn} \times \text{weight in kg}}{2}$$

This is then given using the following formula:

- In the first 12 hours, 3 sets of fluid are given, each over 4 hours
- In the second 12-hour period, 2 sets of fluid are given, each over 6 hours
- In the final 12 hours 1 set of fluid is given

Example

An 80 kg patient with 20% burns would need the following:

$$\frac{20\% \times 80 \text{ kg}}{2} = 800mL$$

- 800mL per 4 hours for the first 12 hours
- 800mL per 6 hours for the second 12 hours
- 800mL for the last 12 hours
- Total fluid = 4800mL in the first 36 hours post-injury

It is important to remember that the calculations use the time of the injury as the starting point, not the time the patient first gets treatment. This may mean that the first quantity of fluid is given very quickly—if a patient takes 3 hours to reach the hospital the initial fluid bolus (using the Parkland formula) would be given over 5 hours. In the example given the rate would be 1280mL/hour.

Regardless of the formula used it must be remembered that they are only guidelines. Close monitoring of the urine output must be maintained to ensure output is at least 1–2mL/kg.

:☢: Inhalation injury

Inhalation injury and the resulting respiratory complications are the main causes of fatality following a burn injury. In any patient who presents with a burn, or who has been exposed to extreme heat, it is essential to immediately assess the airway and to initiate treatment if required.

Key signs and symptoms
- Facial burns
- Burns to the mouth
- Singeing of nasal hair
- Soot in nostrils or in mouth
- Evidence of airway obstruction : wheeze, hoarseness, stridor
- Bronchospasm
- Hypoxia
- Pulmonary oedema

Key history and assessment
- Obtain accurate history of the event(s)
- Ascertain the mechanism of injury
- Check for associated injuries: secondary survey
- Assess the extent and depth of the burn injury

Key observations and findings
- Pulse: tachycardia—pain/fluid loss
- Pulse oximetry: may be difficult to obtain
- Respiratory rate:
  - tachypnoea
  - dyspnoea
  - noisy breathing—suggests airway obstruction
- BP: hypotension—suggests severe fluid loss

Key investigations
- ECG
- XRs
  - CXR
  - cervical spine XR if any risk of a neck injury
- Laboratory investigations:
  - blood gases
  - FBC
  - U&E
  - glucose
  - group and save
  - check carboxyhaemoglobin

Key actions and treatment
- Airway, breathing, and circulation
- Urgent review by experienced doctor
- Refer to anaesthetist if airway involvement is suspected
- Give 100% humidified O_2
- IV access—2 large-bore cannula
- Fluid resuscitation using a recognized formula

- Cardiac monitoring
- Regular recording of vital signs plus pulse oximetry
- Check peak flow rate if possible
- Give salbutamol if there is bronchospasm
- Analgesia: morphine titrated to pain
- Elevate head and chest by 20–30° to reduce neck and chest oedema
- In rare cases escharotomy may be necessary if burn is circumferential to the neck or chest. This is a specialist procedure
- Check tetanus prophylaxis status
- Dress wounds
- Urinary catheter and hourly urine measurement
- NG tube
- Refer to specialist burns unit for admission
- Consider the psychological impact on the patient and their family
- Keep the patient informed of management plan
- Consider the risk of CO or cyanide poisoning

:⚙: Chemical burns

Chemical burns occur most frequently in the workplace. Anyone working with hazardous chemicals should have access to a Control of Substances Hazardous to Health (COSHH) datasheet which provides details of the substance and of the potential health hazards. The amount of tissue damage which occurs depends on the substance involved and the contact time, causing progressive damage until irrigated or neutralized. Injuries can be complicated by systemic absorption.

Chemical burns may involve acids or alkalis. Acids cause proteins to coagulate and thereby limit penetration whereas alkaline substances may continue to penetrate causing deep-tissue injuries unless removed.

Key signs and symptoms
- Localized tissue damage

Key history and assessment
- Time of incident
- Length of contact time
- Chemicals involved
- What first aid measures have already been taken
- Information from COSHH datasheet if available

Key observations and findings
- Baseline pulse, BP, respiratory rate

Key actions and treatment
- *Ensure personal safety*
- Irrigate with copious amounts of water for at least 20min
- 12-lead ECG
- Cardiac monitor
- Vital signs
- Check U&Es
- Analgesia according to pain score
- Obtain specialist advice if required

Cement
On contact with water, the alkaline lime in cement starts to cause tissue damage. Problems occur as people often don't notice due to working conditions and therefore a prolonged contact time occurs, resulting in a deep burn injury. If contact with cement powder occurs then removal by dry brushing is recommended. If a burn is already present then irrigate with water until all traces of cement are removed.

Hydrofluoric acid
Key signs and symptoms
- Intense pain
- Severe tissue damage
- Visible damage may not occur for up to 24 hours

Key history and assessment
- History of contact with hydrofluoric acid—used in the process of glass etching

Key observations and findings
- Pulse
- Respiratory rate
- BP
- Cardiac monitoring
- 12-lead ECG

Key investigations
- U&E
- Serum calcium: severe hypocalcaemia leading to cardiac arrest may occur

Key actions and treatment
- Immediate irrigation required
- Application of calcium gluconate gel
- Pain relief
- Refer for senior medical opinion

Circumferential burns

Any burn encircling the chest wall, neck, limb, or digit may impair breathing or circulation. All circumferential burns should be assessed by a senior clinician. Full thickness burns may require escharotomy which should only be done under specialist supervision.

☼ Electrical burns

The amount of damage caused by an electric shock is more dependant upon the current and contact time than the voltage. Low voltage shocks with high current should not be dismissed lightly. Low voltage is considered to be between 100–240V and is found in domestic household supplies. High voltage is anything >500V and is found in industrial supplies, power lines, railway lines, and lightning. The current follows the path of least resistance through the body. This is often via blood vessels or nerves. It is important to realise the even the smallest of entry wounds can overlie a deep full thickness burn and significant internal injury. Cardiac arrhythmias and respiratory arrest may also occur.

Key signs and symptoms
- Entry and exit wounds
- Muscle tetany
- Associated flash burns
- Altered level of consciousness

Key history and assessment
- Type of current:
  - alternating current—increased risk of arrhythmia, risk of patient being thrown from the electrical source
  - direct current—causes muscle contractions which may make it difficult for the patient to let go thereby increasing the contact time and deep burns
- Voltage involved:
  - low voltage—may cause serious deep burn injuries
  - high voltage—may cause associated injuries, may cause flash burns, igniting clothing and causing thermal skin burns as well as internal electrical burns
- Contact time
- Entry point: often very small but with a serious deep burn injury underneath
- Exit point:
  - not always obvious
  - check the first place likely to be in contact with the ground, back of the head, base of spine, tip of shoulder etc.
  - if present then consider a burn pathway between the contact point and the exit
- Associated injuries:
  - musculoskeletal injuries may result from falls etc.
  - fractures or dislocations as a result of extreme muscle spasm

Key observations and findings
- Pulse
- Respiratory rate
- O_2 saturation
- Neurological observations
- Distal circulation and sensation

- Monitor urinary output hourly
- Observe urine for myoglobinuria—presence of myogloblin, a muscle protein in the urine—which presents as darkened urine

Key investigations
- Cardiac monitoring
- 12-lead ECG
- FBC
- U&Es
- Creatine kinase: indicates muscle damage
- Urinalysis for blood

Key actions and treatment
- ABC assessment
- O_2
- IV fluids may be required
- Give analgesia according to pain score
- Check for and treat wounds
- Patients should be referred for an experienced medical opinion prior to discharge
- Asymptomatic patients may be discharged home
- Others will require admission for observation and monitoring

:✪: Facial burns

The majority of facial burns are the result of flame flashback or high-pressure steam. These result in very short contact times and therefore most are superficial injuries. Once the risk of an inhalation injury has been excluded, superficial burns to the face can be managed without admission to hospital. A number of different treatments are used without any one appearing to be more effective than any other. The main principle is to keep the face clean and moist. Facial burns which receive no treatment appear to do as well as those which have ointment or lotions applied. If ointment is required then simple soft paraffin ointment is as effective as anything.

Any burn which affects the mouth, eyes, cartilage of the ears or nose should be referred to a specialist centre.

① Hand burns

The aim of treating burns to the hand is to prevent infection and maintain mobility. With the exception of small superficial burns which do not involve joints, specialist advice should be sought. Local guidelines for dressings should be followed.

① Perineal burns

Any burn involving the perineum requires careful management. Problems include difficulties in applying effective dressings and a high risk of infection. Consideration should be given to admitting these patients to ensure adequate wound management.

① Superficial burns

Although causing no serious long-term problems superficial burns can still be very worrying for patients who may be concerned about pain, scarring, and loss of function. Superficial burns heal within 14 days unless they become infected. Treatment is aimed at managing pain and preventing infection. Following a superficial burn patients should be advised to use sun block over the affected area when outdoors for at least 12 months.

Key signs and symptoms
- Painful
- Red or pink discolouration

Key history and assessment
- Ascertain mechanism of injury
- Contact time
- Note the time since the burn occurred
- Even if the burn is small and superficial, ensure the patient has no risk of inhalation injury
- Tetanus status

Key observations and findings
- Baseline pulse and temperature may be required

Key investigations
- None required

Key actions and treatment
- Provide pain relief:
    - often simple analgesia such as paracetamol 1g is enough to make the pain bearable for the patient
    - Entonox®, 50% O_2 and 50% nitrous oxide may be helpful while first assessing the burn
- Clean and dress the burn according to local guidelines
- Provide clear instructions to the patient on:
    - how to continue caring for the burn
    - what to expect during the healing process
    - how to obtain help if required
    - advice on accident prevention to prevent recurrence

Burn dressings
There has been an ongoing debate about the optimum wound management regimen for burns for many years with no clear consensus emerging. The perfect dressing is one which:
- Act as a barrier to infection
- Provides mechanical protection
- Maintains a moist healing environment
- Removes excess exudates
- Prevents 'strike through' of exudates
- Maintains optimum healing temperature
- Allows gaseous exchange
- Maintains good contact with the healthy skin

- Does not adhere to the damaged tissue
- Is easy to remove without causing any additional trauma
- Is acceptable to the patient
- Non-toxic
- Non-allergenic
- Non-sensitizing

Unfortunately, despite great efforts from manufacturers, the perfect dressing does not yet exist and therefore either a compromise must be made based on the most likely requirements of the wound, or different dressings used for different stages of the healing.

In choosing a dressing, the nurse needs to assess the individual needs of the patient and the type and state of the burn. Wherever possible the choice should be evidence based.

Any blistering should be left intact if at all possible. If the blister is under pressure and likely to burst then it should be drained with a sterile needle and syringe and dressed with a sterile dressing.

⑦ Sunburn

Many people experience the pain and discomfort of sunburn every year with the vast majority self-caring. If the assistance of a healthcare professional is sought it is normally for help with pain relief or blistering.

Key signs and symptoms
- Redness
- Tender to touch
- Pain on movement
- Blistering

Key history and assessment
- Excessive exposure to the sun
- Assess to ensure no evidence of heatstroke
- Use of sun block with appropriate sun protection factor (SPF)

Key observations and findings
- May wish to check temperature if any suspicion of heat stroke

Key investigations
- None required

Key actions and treatment
- Provide simple analgesia
- Advice on fluid intake to prevent dehydration
- Advice on preventive measures

Chest pain

Differential diagnosis

:ⓧ: True emergencies

- Aortic dissection
- Myocardial infarction
- Oesophageal rupture

:ⓧ: Urgent presentations

- Angina
- Blunt trauma
- Chest infection
- Pericarditis
- Pleuritic pain
- Pneumothorax
- Pulmonary embolus

ⓘ Timely assessment

- Anxiety
- Gallbladder disease
- Gastritis
- Gastro-oesophageal reflux disease
- Musculoskeletal pain

☠ Aortic dissection

Aortic dissection can present as severe sudden central chest pain, often radiating to the back. The pain is often described as tearing or ripping and soon accompanied by signs of hypovolaemic shock. Rapid diagnosis and surgical intervention is essential, even then mortality rates are high. The diagnosis may need to be made on the clinical findings alone as the patients condition is to critical to delay while investigations are undertaken.

☐ See Abdominal pain, p.1.

☠ Myocardial infarction

Acute MI (AMI) occurs when there is necrosis of myocardium as the result of an interruption to the coronary blood supply. Most commonly this is caused by atherosclerosis of the coronary artery leading to occlusion by a thrombus. Life-threatening arrhythmias or heart failure can occur as a result.

Key signs and symptoms
- Pain:
  - central, crushing, retrosternal pain
  - lasting >20min despite analgesia
  - commencing at rest
  - radiating to jaw, neck, one or both arms
  - epigastric pain is common with myocardial ischaemia
- Breathlessness
- N&V
- Pallor
- Cold sweats
- Anxiety or 'feeling of impending doom'

Key history and assessment
- Previous MI
- Other cardiac problems
- Hypertension
- Smoker
- Hypercholesterolaemia
- Lack of exercise
- High alcohol intake
- Obese
- Diabetes
- Family history
  - cardiac problems
  - stroke
  - sudden unexplained death

Key observations and findings
- Pulse:
  - usually normal
  - bradycardia may occur with an inferior infarction

- Respiratory rate:
  - usually normal
  - dyspnoea may occur due to left ventricular failure
- BP: hypertension is common

Key investigations

- 12-lead ECG:
  - changes will demonstrate the area of the myocardium that is damaged and the progress of the infarction
  - may be normal in the early stages
  - repeat recordings will be required, these must be dated and timed clearly
- CXR: not routinely required unless the patient is dyspnoeic
- Laboratory tests:
  - troponin: tropT or tropI according to local practice
  - glucose
  - U&Es + serum cholesterol
  - FBC
  - ABGs: if the patient is dyspnoeic

Key actions and treatment

- Immediate medical assessment
- High-flow O_2 via a non-rebreathing mask
- IV access
- Continuous cardiac monitoring due to risk of developing life-threatening arrhythmias
- Aspirin 300mg orally
- IV morphine for pain relief, titrated to the patient's response
- IV anti-emetic if required
- Consider eligibility for thrombolysis or angioplasty
- Treat in a calm controlled manner
- Fast track to coronary care unit (CCU)

Thrombolysis

In AMI thrombolytic drugs break down the thrombus so the blood flow to the heart muscle can be restored. Early restoration of the coronary circulation reduces damage and improves prognosis. Along with clinical symptoms, characteristic changes in the 12-lead ECG (ST segment elevation) provide the most immediate indication of the diagnosis of AMI.

Early administration is vital in providing maximum benefit from thrombolysis. Treatment should be commenced as soon as possible after the onset of symptoms. In England and Wales the aim is to provide thrombolysis within 60min of a patient contacting a healthcare professional. The main risk of thrombolysis is haemorrhagic stroke which occurs in 1 in 100 patients. Bleeding can also occur anywhere in the GI tract.

Contraindications:

- Recent:
  - haemorrhage
  - trauma
  - surgery
  - stroke

- Bleeding disorders
- Very high BP: >180mmHg systolic

Thrombolytic agents

Streptokinase

- Administered as an IV infusion
- Can be used up to 12 hours after the onset of symptoms
- Frequently causes hypotension—do not use if patient hypotensive
- Can cause allergic reactions
- Patients develop anti-streptococcal antibodies, therefore it can only be given once in a patient's lifetime
- Does not require the use of heparin

rt-PA (alteplase)

- Initial IV bolus injection followed by infusion
- Can be used up to 12 hours after onset of symptoms
- Heparin also needs to be given

Reteplase

- Two IV bolus injections 30min apart
- Can be used up to 12 hours after symptoms first start
- Heparin also needs to be given

Tenecteplase

- Single IV bolus injection
- Can be used up to 12 hours after onset of symptoms
- Heparin also needs to be given

For those agents which require the administration of heparin, this is given as an IV bolus injection prior to the thrombolysis followed by an IV infusion.

Primary percutaneous coronary intervention (PCI), which is an invasive procedure designed to open the occluded artery, is an alternative to thrombolysis in those hospitals which have the appropriate facilities.

☹ Oesophageal rupture

A rupture of the oesophagus allows food or fluids to leak into the chest and causes severe lung problems. The onset of signs and symptoms depends on the cause and location of the rupture. Damage to the intra-thoracic oesophagus can result in severe symptoms within minutes.

Key signs and symptoms
- Retrosternal pain progressing to severe epigastric pain
- Pain worse on swallowing
- N&V
- Surgical emphysema in the neck
- The combination of vomiting, chest pain, and surgical emphysema occurs in about 50% of patients and is known as Mackler's triad. It is characteristic of the diagnosis
- Haematemesis
- Pyrexia
- Dyspnoea
- Cyanosis

Key history and assessment
History needs to be focused on finding a cause for the condition. These include:
- Intubation
- Recent endoscopy
- Blunt or penetrating trauma to the chest or neck
- Ingestion of corrosive chemicals
- Swallowing a foreign object
- Pre-existing oesophageal ulceration
- Oesophageal cancer
- Forceful vomiting

Key observations and findings
Depends on the location, cause, and time since the incident. May be little to find at first but can rapidly progress to demonstrate clinical signs of infection and/or shock:
- Tachycardia
- Tachypnoea
- Hypotension
- Pyrexia

Key investigations
- CXR:
  - air or fluid in the pleural cavity
  - mediastinal emphysema

Key actions and treatment
- Refer to surgical team for urgent assessment. The vast majority of patients will require urgent surgery
- Nil-by-mouth
- Continual vital signs and cardiac monitoring
- IV analgesia as required

- O_2 therapy
- IV fluids as required to maintain BP
- May be considered for conservative management if:
  - early diagnosis
  - patient has not eaten anything since the injury
  - no distal obstruction by tumor or stricture
  - no signs of any acute illness other than pain
  - no signs of sepsis
- Requires broad-spectrum antibiotics according to local guidelines

:O: Angina

Angina is a symptom of inadequate coronary blood flow to the myocardium resulting in chest pain. It is most commonly a symptom of coronary artery disease, although it can occur in anaemic patients who have insufficient red blood cells to carry O_2 to the myocardium.

Types of angina
- Stable:
  - frequency and severity of attacks are well controlled and unchanged
  - caused by an increase in myocardial O_2 demand during exercise, exertion, or stress
- Unstable:
  - pain increasing in frequency, severity, and duration
  - occurring at rest
  - pain lasting >20min

Key signs and symptoms
- Central chest pain
- May range from mild discomfort to severe pain
- May be described as 'tightness' rather than pain
- May radiate to the jaw and/or the arms
- May be exercise related
- May be relieved by rest—stable angina
- Epigastric discomfort is a common symptom of ischaemia

Key history and assessment
- If known history of angina, what is different about this episode
- Is pain eased with glyceryl trinitrate (GTN), O_2 or rest
- Known hypertension
- Smoker or ex-smoker
- Obese
- Sedentary lifestyle
- High blood cholesterol
- Diabetes
- Family history of male relative <55 or female relative <65 with heart disease

Key observations and findings
- Pulse, rate, rhythm
- Respiratory rate
- BP: both arms
- Location, duration, and nature of pain
- Relationship to exertion
- Pallor or cyanosis
- Nausea or vomiting

Key investigations
- 12-lead ECG
- FBC
- U&Es
- Glucose
- Cardiac enzymes

Key actions and treatment
- Pain relief:
  - sublingual GTN 0.3-1mg
  - high-flow O_2 via a non-rebreather mask
  - may require IV opiates
- Aspirin 300mg
- IV access
- Cardiac monitoring and regular recording of vital signs
- Refer to medical team for further assessment

:⚙: Blunt trauma

Blunt chest wall trauma is relatively common as an isolated injury or in conjunction with multiple trauma. Management is focused first on identifying any potential serious underlying injuries through a primary survey.

First and second rib fractures

Any fractures to the first or second ribs should raise awareness of the potential for underlying major internal injuries.

Fractures of ribs 4–10

These are the most common blunt chest injury. There may be significant underlying injuries depending on the mechanism and forces involved. These injuries tend to be more problematic in the elderly and those with chronic respiratory problems.

Fractures of ribs 8–12

Need to exclude underlying abdominal injury.

Key signs and symptoms
- Chest pain on inspiration
- Patient reluctant to breathe deeply due to pain
- Localized tenderness on palpation
- Crepitus over fracture(s)

Key history and assessment
- History of known traumatic event
- History of chest pain with no known traumatic event but following high risk activity:
  - contact sport
  - recent alcohol intoxication
- No associated cardiac signs or symptoms
- No cardiac risk factors

Key observations and findings
- Pulse usually within normal range
- Respirations may demonstrate an altered pattern of breathing as the patient attempts to control respiratory pain by modifying breathing
- Temperature: normal
- BP: within normal parameters
- Pulse oximetry should be recorded
- Any abnormality in vital signs should raise suspicion of an underlying serious injury—such as pneumothorax

Key investigations
- CXR
- ABGs if concerned about inadequate respirations
- 12-lead ECG

Key actions and treatment
- If acutely short of breath give supplementary O_2
- Pain control:
  - simple oral analgesia may be adequate for isolated fractures
  - advise the patient these will reduce, not remove the pain
  - warn the patient that the pain may continue for several weeks
  - opiates and NSAIDs may be required for more severe pain
- Encourage deep breathing while splinting painful area
- Early mobilization
- Patients with single rib fractures whose pain can be managed with oral analgesia and who are showing no signs of respiratory distresses may be discharged
- Any signs of respiratory distress, pain management problems, or underlying injury will require admission

Flail segment

Three or more consecutive ribs, fractured in two or more places, will produce an unstable area in the chest wall which moves independently of the rest of the rib cage. A large amount of force is required to cause this injury and there is often underlying damage.

Sternal fractures

The majority of sternal fractures are the result of high impact forces such as road traffic collisions (seat belt injury). Up to 70% of patients have other injuries, including head trauma, rib fractures, and limb fractures. Mortality is low from sternal fracture unless an associated injury is present. Sternal fracture can also be a side effect of cardiopulmonary resuscitation.

Key signs and symptoms
- Depends on severity of injury
- Chest pain
- Localized tenderness
- Bruising occurs in <50% of cases
- Pain on inspiration
- Dyspnoea: consider pneumothorax

Key history and assessment
- History of trauma, mechanism of injury, time of injury
- Visual assessment of wounds and extent of bruising
- Palpation may reveal crepitus or step defect in sternum
- Auscultation to ensure breath sounds equal and no underlying lung damage
- Assess pain level

Key observations and findings
- Pulse rate: rhythm and volume
- Respirations: rate, depth, pattern
- Pulse oximetry should be recorded
- BP
- Observe chest symmetry and extent of expansion

Key investigations

- 12-lead ECG
- CXR and sternal views to determine extent and location of fracture
- ABGs if patient has respiratory distress

Key actions and treatment

- Ensure airway is patent and breathing is adequate
- Give supplementary O_2
- Cardiac monitoring until cardiac injury excluded
- Analgesia, managing pain is key to the treatment of sternal fractures:
  - should be based on patient response
  - oral NSAIDs
  - consider opiates, oral or IV as required
- Exclude associated injuries
- May require admitting for pain management
- If no complications present and the pain can be managed the patient may be discharged
- No external splinting or bandaging should be applied as these reduce chest expansion and restrict breathing
- Advise to avoid lifting, carrying, or other activities which involve the pectoral and shoulder girdle muscles

:O: Chest infection

Patients may present with chest pain, but this is associated with respiratory signs and symptoms, pre-existing chronic obstructive pulmonary disease (COPD) or obvious signs of infection. It is important, however, to exclude a cardiac cause as this may coexist with a respiratory problem.

📖 See Shortness of breath, p.367.

:O: Pericarditis

The heart is surrounded by two membranous layers, the visceral pericardium and the parietal pericardium. Between the two is a potential space containing pericardial fluid. Pericarditis occurs when one or both of these membranes becomes inflamed. Most commonly the inflammation is viral in origin, although it can be caused by various agents including bacteria, invasive cancer, and trauma. It may also occur as a complication of renal failure. However, the majority of cases are idiopathic. Although it can affect people of all ages it is most common in men between the ages of 20–50 years.

Key signs and symptoms
- Central or left-sided chest pain:
  - may radiate to the neck or shoulder
  - may be positional
  - may be affected by breathing
- Fever
- Shortness of breath, worse on lying down

Key history and assessment
- Recent or current infection:
  - viral
  - bacterial
- MI within the last 4 months—Dressler's syndrome
- Malignancy
- Uraemia
- Trauma
- Hypothyroidism

Key observations and findings
- Baseline temperature, pulse, and respiratory rate
- Sinus tachycardia may be present
- Pulse oximetry

Key investigations
- FBC: raised white cell count indicative of infection
- U&Es/C-reactive protein (CRP)
- ECG:
  - concave, saddle-shaped ST segment elevation
  - changes are present in all chest leads
- Blood cultures if bacterial infection suspected

- Echocardiogram
- Thyroid function tests (TFTs)

Key actions and treatment
- Refer to medical team
- Analgesia:
  - opiates may be needed in the acute phase
  - NSAIDs may help treat underlying inflammation
- Bed rest
- Cardiac monitor
- Regular recording of vital signs
- May require O_2 therapy
- Steroids may be required of the pain does not settle
- Antibiotics if required
- Treat underlying cause if found

:☼: Pleuritic pain

Inflammation of the pleural membranes covering the lungs presents with short sharp chest pain which is worse on inhalation or coughing. It is accompanied with pyrexia and shallow breathing in an attempt to control the pain. The usual cause is a viral infection, although it can occur as a side effect of pneumonia or a pulmonary embolus. Rarely, it is an autoimmune condition.

📖 See Shortness of breath, p.367.

:☼: Pneumothorax

Pneumothorax may occur following blunt or penetrating trauma. It can, however, happen spontaneously in tall, slender young men or secondary to underlying chronic chest disease. Presentation may be with a sudden onset of unilateral pleuritic chest pain. The development of a tension pneumothorax is life threatening, as a one-way valve is created allowing air into the pleural space each time the patient takes a breath, but preventing this escaping on expiration.

📖 See Shortness of breath, p.367.

☼ Pulmonary embolus

Although normally presenting with sudden onset of breathlessness pulmonary embolism (PE) may be accompanied by sharp, central chest pain which is pleuritic in nature. It can be difficult to diagnose and should be considered particularly in patients who have had a long period of immobilization, a history of previous PE/deep vein thrombosis (DVT), or in women who have recently given birth.

📖 See Shortness of breath, p.367.

① Anxiety

Chest pain is a common symptom in patients suffering from anxiety. Cardiac reasons and other physical pathology for the pain should be excluded before consideration is given to anxiety as a cause.

Key signs and symptoms
- Chest pain
- Hyperventilation, dizziness, and paraesthesia
- Psychological distress
- Palpitations
- Statements about inability to breathe

Key history and assessment
- History of previous anxiety disorders
- Sleep disturbance
- Identifiable recent stressors, close bereavement, unemployment, divorce, sudden change in personal circumstances

Key observations and findings
- Usually normal
- Tachycardia may be present
- Hyperventilation

Key investigations
- 12-lead ECG: no abnormalities
- Cardiac monitoring: shows sinus rhythm

Key actions and treatment
- Reassure the patient that the pain is not cardiac
- Ask directly about recent feelings of panic and life stresses
- Consider follow up in primary care

① Gallbladder disease

Inflammation of the gallbladder, cholecystitis, and gallstones can all present with pain which radiates into the chest. It is often accompanied by pyrexia and N&V and may demonstrate a relationship to meals.

📖 See Abdominal pain, p.1.

① Gastritis

Gastritis and peptic ulceration can occasionally present with chest pain. The pain is described as burning, but may be felt as a tightness or heaviness. There is a relationship to food, with light meals often relieving the pain, but alcohol or caffeine making it worse. It may be relived with antacids and 12-lead ECG is normal. *It is vital to exclude cardiac causes for a patient presenting with 'indigestion'.*

📖 See Abdominal pain, p.1.

① Gastro-oesophageal reflux disease

Gastro-oesophageal reflux disease (GORD) occurs when gastric acid refluxes into the oesophagus. It is commonly referred to as indigestion or heartburn, but can be mistaken as acute cardiac pain. Patients present with central chest pain directly beneath the sternum. Often this is described as a burning pain, but sometimes it is felt as a heaviness or tightness. It may be accompanied by burping or an acid taste in the mouth. There is often a relationship to eating and the pain is worse on bending over or lying down. 12-lead ECG is normal and the symptoms can be relieved with antacids. More serious is the risk of patients dismissing cardiac pain as indigestion or heartburn and ignoring the onset of symptoms. *It is vital to exclude cardiac causes for a patient presenting with 'indigestion'.*

📖 See Abdominal pain, p.1.

⊙ Musculoskeletal pain

Musculoskeletal pain in the chest wall is common, particularly following excessive physical exertion or trauma. It may also occur in patients with rheumatic disorders. The majority of patients can be managed with simple oral analgesia. It is important to exclude cardiac problems and other underlying serious pathology.

Key signs and symptoms
- Deep aching pain
- Difficult to localize
- Worse on movement
- Not radiating

Key history and assessment
- History of trauma
- History of recent physical activity
- History of recent cough
- Pain worse on palpation of injured area

Key observations and findings
- Pulse: normal or slight tachycardia due to pain or infection
- BP: normal
- Temperature: normal unless associated infection
- Respirations may demonstrate an altered pattern due to pain
- SpO$_2$ should be >97%
- Examine chest wall for any signs of trauma or inflammation

Key investigations
- None normally required
- ABGs: if any signs of compromised breathing
- CXR: if underlying lung injury/pathology or rib fractures suspected
- 12-lead ECG: if any indication of a cardiac problem

Key actions and treatment
- Pain relief
- Advice on deep breathing exercises to prevent chest infection
- Treat any underlying condition

Collapse

Differential diagnosis

☻ True emergencies
- Anaphylaxis
- Cardiac arrest
- Fitting
- Obstructed airway
- Shock
- Hypovolaemia
- Cardiogenic shock
- Septic shock
- Neurogenic shock
- Unconscious patient

☼ Urgent presentations
- Cardiac arrhythmias
- Hypoglycaemia
- Hypothermia
- Myocardial infarction
- Poisoning
- Stroke/transient ischaemic attack

① Timely assessment
- Vaso-vagal syncope

Introduction

The term 'collapse' covers a range of conditions, from simple faints to cardiac arrest. Specifically the term refers to the inability of a patient to maintain an upright posture. Initial assessment is required in all patients in order to determine whether the event is life threatening. A detailed history of the event from the patient or witness is essential. All nurses should be competent in the provision of basic life support.

☠ Anaphylaxis

Anaphylaxis is a severe allergic reaction. Histamine release causes tissue swelling, airway constriction, circulatory collapse, and sometimes death. Immediate medical intervention is required.

📖 See Allergy, p.31.

☠ Cardiac arrest

Key signs and symptoms
- Collapse
- Unconsciousness
- Absence of pulse
- Absence of respiration
- Cyanosis

Key history and assessment
- Sudden collapse

Key observations and findings
- Absence of respiration
- Pulseless
- Unresponsive

Key investigations
- No investigations required until resuscitation is commenced
- Cardiac monitor to check for:
  - shockable rhythms: ventricular fibrillation (VF) or ventricular tachycardia (VT)
  - non-shockable rhythms: asystole or pulseless electrical activity (PEA)
- ABGs
- If resuscitation is successful:
  - 12-lead ECG
  - U&Es, cardiac enzymes

Key actions and treatment
- Ensure the area is safe
- Check responsiveness
- Call for help
- Check and clear the airway
- Assess for signs of life, breathing, and circulation
- Summon resuscitation team/dial 999. If you are alone you should leave the patient in order to do this
- Commence life support according to Resuscitation Council guidelines
- Ensure care of relatives and family

☢ Fitting

Alternatively referred to as convulsions or seizures, fits often present as an emergency due to the sudden onset and anxiety which they cause in witnesses. Fits occur as a result of sudden disorganized electrical activity in the brain. The effects on the individual will depend on the area and extent of the brain involved. There are many causes which can be classified into five main groups:

- Cerebral irritation—haemorrhage, infection, neoplasm
- Metabolic disorders—hypoglycemia, low sodium
- Drug/alcohol withdrawal
- Idiopathic
- Pseudo-seizures

During a seizure the only intervention required is to prevent further injury occurring. Do not try to restrain the patient or place anything into their mouth. As soon as the seizure stops place the patient into the recovery position and be aware they may be confused during recovery.

📖 See Fits, p.225.

☠ Obstructed airway

Key signs and symptoms
- Respiratory distress:
  - increased respiratory effort
  - use of accessory muscles
  - tracheal tug
  - intercostal recession
  - noisy breathing or stridor
  - colour change, pallor, or cyanosis
- Respiratory arrest

Key history and assessment
- Level of consciousness
- Assess chest movement
- Listen for breath sounds
- Check for tracheal deviation—tension pneumothorax
- Relevant history:
  - trauma
  - asthma
  - COPD
  - inhaled FB
  - croup
  - epiglottitis
  - smoke inhalation
  - allergic reaction

Key observations and findings
- Respiratory rate: tachypnoea, dyspnoea, apnoea
- Pulse: tachycardia
- BP
- SpO_2: <94% on air

Key investigations
- Airway intervention should be undertaken (if required) before any investigations
- FBC, U&E, ABGs
- ECG
- CXR
- Other investigations relevant to underlying problem

Key actions and treatment
- Call for immediate help
- Check airway, remove any obvious obstruction if possible
- Give high-flow O_2
- Maintain airway
- Assist breathing via bag-valve-mask if required
- Cardiac monitoring
- Regularly monitor vital signs
- IV access
- Definitive treatment for underlying problem

☠ Shock

A clinical syndrome characterized by a lack of adequate tissue perfusion. The O_2 and nutritional needs of the cells are not met and the cells and organs are unable to function properly. If untreated, cell and organ failure ensues, followed by death.

Classification

- Hypovolaemic: fluid loss—blood, plasma, diarrhoea, vomiting
- Cardiogenic:
  - post MI
  - arrhythmias
  - cardiac tamponade
  - tension pneumothorax
- Septic: overwhelming bacterial infection
- Neurogenic: hypotension and bradycardia associated with cervical or high thoracic spinal cord injury

☠ Hypovolaemia

This is the commonest cause of shock. It occurs as a result of fluid loss which may be internal or external. The circulating blood volume is reduced to the point where vital organs can not be adequately perfused. The loss may follow haemorrhage, extensive burns, or diarrhoea.

Key signs and symptoms

- Obvious signs of bleeding
- Increased thirst
- Cool and clammy skin
- Pallor
- Delayed capillary refill
- Reduced urinary output
- Altered level of consciousness, confusion, aggression, drowsiness
- Collapse

Key history and assessment

- Identify the source of the fluid loss
- History of trauma
- Obvious signs of haemorrhage
- Aortic aneurysm
- Early pregnancy: ectopic
- Vomiting or diarrhoea
- Burns
- Polyuria: hyperglycaemia

Key observations and findings

- Hypovolaemia is classified depending on the observations of the patient, see Table 12.1

Table 12.1 Classification of hypovolaemia (based on a 70kg patient)

Grade	I	II	III	IV
Volume lost	750mL (15%)	1.5L (30%)	2L (40%)	2.5L (>40%)
Urine output	Normal	20–30mL/hour	<20mL/hour	No output
Pulse	Normal	Tachycardia <120	Tachycardia >120	
BP	Normal	Postural hypotension	Hypotension	Unrecordable
Pulse pressure	Normal	Decreased	Decreased	Unrecordable
Capillary return	Normal	Normal	Decreased	Markedly decreased
Mental status	Normal	Mildly anxious	Anxious and confused	Confused, lethargic

Key investigations

- Blood glucose
- ABGs
- Group and save or cross match depending on clinical condition
- FBC, U&Es
- 12-lead ECG
- CXR
- CT or ultrasound if required to identify bleeding

Key actions and treatment

- Immediate medical support required
- Ensure a clear airway is maintained
- High-level O_2 via a non-rebreathing mask
- Lie patient flat (if possible) and elevate the legs
- Continuous cardiac monitoring
- Insert 2 large-bore cannulae
- Commence IV fluids according to local policy
- Regular recording of vital signs
- Catheterize, hourly urine output monitoring
- Definitive treatment to prevent further fluid loss

☠ Cardiogenic shock

This occurs following a cardiac event which results in the heart being unable to circulate sufficient blood to the vital organs. The causes may include electrical conduction problems, myocardial ischaemia, or valve disease. Adequate circulating volume is present but the flow is reduced.

Key signs and symptoms
- Collapse
- Cold and clammy skin
- Poor peripheral perfusion
- Pallor or cyanosis
- Mental impairment

Key history and assessment
- Previous cardiac problems
- Pre-existing medical problem(s)
- MI

Key observations and findings
- Respiratory rate: tachypnoea
- Pulse: tachycardia, weak
- Delayed capillary refill
- BP: hypotension
- SpO_2 <94%
- GCS <15
- Reduced urinary output

Key investigations
- Blood gases
- FBC, U&Es
- Cardiac enzymes
- Blood glucose
- 12-lead ECG
- CXR

Key actions and treatment
- Immediate medical support required
- Ensure a clear airway is maintained
- High-flow O_2 via a non-rebreathing mask
- Continuous cardiac monitoring
- Insert 2 large-bore cannulae
- Commence IV fluids cautiously
- Regular recording of vital signs
- Catheterize, hourly urine output monitoring
- Ensure reversible causes are corrected e.g. cardiac tamponade, pulmonary embolus, tension pneumothorax

:☀: Septic shock

Caused by overwhelming bacterial infection. Hypotension and hypovolaemia occur.

Key signs and symptoms
- Sweats, chills, or rigors
- Fever
- Breathlessness
- Headache
- Confusion
- Obvious site of infection

Key history and assessment
- History of recent infection
- Pneumonia
- Intra-abdominal sepsis
- UTI
- Skin and soft tissue infection
- Meningitis

Key observations and findings
- Respiratory rate: tachypnoea, dyspnoea
- Temperature: pyrexia >38°C or hypothermia <35.6°C
- BP: hypotensive
- Pulse: tachycardia with bounding peripheral pulses
- SpO_2: <94% on air
- GCS <15
- Oliguria

Key investigations
- ABGs
- FBC, U&E, blood cultures
- Culture of sputum, urine, wound and throat swabs as appropriate
- 12-lead ECG
- CXR
- Ultrasound or CT of abdomen if appropriate

Key actions and observations
- Immediate medical support required
- Ensure a clear airway is maintained
- High-flow O_2 via a non-rebreathing mask
- Continuous cardiac monitoring
- Insert 2 large-bore cannulae
- Commence IV fluids
- Regular recording of vital signs
- Catheterize, hourly urine output monitoring
- Antibiotic therapy according to local guidelines
- Antipyretics
- Maintain patient comfort with regular bedding changes
- Frequent position changes or air mattress to maintain tissue viability

☠: **Neurogenic shock**

Damage to the central nervous system can result in sudden loss of sympathetic nerve supply to the blood vessels. A decrease in peripheral vascular resistance follows along with a drop in BP. Most commonly this results from trauma to the spine or following a head injury.

Key signs and symptoms
- Collapse
- Warm and dry peripheral skin
- Priapism may occur
- Limb weakness, loss of sensation
- Respiratory distress

Key history and assessment
- History of trauma, especially head or neck injury
- Patient may have other serious injuries
- Check for other causes of hypotension e.g., blood loss
- Pre-existing medical problems
- Local pain and tenderness over site of injury
- Sensory deficit
- Reduced limb tone
- Assess reflexes for flaccidity or arreflexia
- Reduced anal tone
- Diaphragmatic breathing

Key observations and findings
- Pulse: bradycardia
- BP: hypotension
- Temperature
- Respiratory rate: tachypnoea, dyspnoea

Key investigations
- FBC, U&E, ABGs
- 12-lead ECG
- CXR, cervical spine and pelvis XRs
- CT may be required

Key actions and observations
- Immediate medical support required
- Ensure a clear airway is maintained
- High flow O_2 via a non-rebreathing mask
- Continuous cardiac monitoring
- If head or back injury:
  - immobilize head and neck in neutral position
  - apply hard collar and support with sandbags and tape
- Insert 2 large-bore cannulae
- Commence IV fluids
- Regular recording of vital signs
- Catheterize, hourly urine output monitoring
- Maintain patient comfort with regular bedding changes

- Frequent position changes or air mattress to maintain tissue viability
- Insert a NG tube to prevent gastric distension
- Log roll to examine the back
- Keep patient warm and covered to reduce risk of hypothermia
- Pressure area care for tissue viability

☣ **Unconscious patient**

Key signs and symptoms
- Unresponsive

Key history and assessment
- Obtain history from any witnesses
- Assess potential causes:
  - poisoning, alcohol, or drugs
  - hypoglycaemia
  - stroke
  - head injury
  - post-ictal state
  - subarachnoid haemorrhage
  - respiratory failure
  - hypotension
  - cardiac arrhythmias
  - MI
  - hypothermia
  - hypovolaemia
  - overwhelming infection

Key observations and findings
- Pulse, respiratory rate, BP: may be normal or abnormal depending on the reason for the condition
- All must be recorded at frequent regular intervals, including the GCS and pulse oximetry

Key investigations
- Blood glucose
- ABGs
- FBC, U&Es
- 12-lead ECG
- Cardiac enzymes, if appropriate
- Urinalysis
- CXR
- CT scan if intracranial pathology suspected

Key actions and treatment
- Immediate medical assessment
- Ensure a clear airway
- Maintain airway
- Ensure breathing and circulation present
- If trauma is suspected, protect the cervical spine with a semi-rigid collar
- Give high-flow O_2 via a non-rebreathing mask
- Continuous cardiac monitoring
- Frequently monitor vital signs including GCS
- Pulse oximetry
- Cannulation
- IV fluids as required
- Check for medi-alert bracelet

- Check for signs of trauma
- Obtain history from paramedics/relatives/GP
- Treat any identifiable causes of unconsciousness
- Pressure area care
- Explanations must be given to the patient regardless of level of response

⊙ Cardiac arrhythmias

A number of cardiac arrhythmias may cause a patient to suddenly collapse. VF or pulseless VT result in cardiac arrest and require resuscitation. Others which briefly interrupt cardiac output can cause collapse and a brief period of unconsciousness. Patients require urgent medical assessment.

📖 See Palpitations, p.327.

⊙ Hypoglycaemia

Hypoglycaemia should be considered in any patient who suffers a sudden collapse.

All patients should have blood glucose recorded at the earliest opportunity once the airway, breathing, and circulation has been assessed and managed. If the blood glucose is <3mmol/L the patient will require additional glucose. If conscious this can be in the form of a glucose drink followed by complex carbohydrate (e.g. a sandwich). If the patient has a reduced conscious level then a preparation such as a glucose gel which can be absorbed by the buccal mucosa may be used. If unconscious, 50mL 50% glucose IV will be required.

📖 See Diabetes, p.157.

:⚙: Hypothermia

Hypothermia occurs when the core body temperature drops below 35°C. People with conditions affecting their capacity to respond to changes in temperature such as hypothyroidism, substance misuse, or stroke are at higher risk. Older people have a higher incidence due to poor mobility, malnutrition, polypharmacy, and pre-existing medical conditions. Anyone who has fallen and spent time on the floor should be considered to be at risk. Severe hypothermia may mimic death.

Key signs and symptoms

- Mild 32–35°C:
  - shivering
  - cold to touch
  - lethargy
  - pallor
- Moderate 30–32°C:
  - uncontrollable shivering
  - altered consciousness level
  - weakness
- Severe <30°C:
  - not shivering
  - dilated pupils
  - muscle rigidity
  - unconscious
  - cardiac arrest may occur

Key history and assessment

- Assessment is based on physical findings and observations
- Signs of malnutrition
- Exposure due to inadequate clothing, heating, or near drowning
- Current medications
- Evidence of substance misuse
- Endocrine abnormalities
- Mobility problems

Key observations and findings

- Core temperature: <35°C
- Pulse: weak and thready, bradycardia
- BP: hypotension, may be unrecordable
- Respirations: bradypnoea, shallow, irregular

Key investigations

- Check core (rectal) temperature
- Blood glucose
- ABGs
- FBC, U&E, clotting screen, amylase, blood cultures
- 12-lead ECG
- Urinalysis
- CXR

Key actions and observations
- Medical assessment required
- Aim of treatment is to stabilize and rewarm
- Patients should be handled gently as there is a risk of causing cardiac arrhythmias or arrest
- Do not vigorously rub patients
- Mild hypothermia:
  - remove wet or cold clothes
  - rewarm passively with blankets and warm environment
  - cover patient's head to reduce heat loss
  - warm drinks if able to swallow, alcohol should not be given as it lowers temperature.
  - if able to eat give food
  - If mobile encourage movement
- Moderate/severe hypothermia:
  - warm humidified O_2
  - establish IV access
  - correct hypoglycaemia
  - urinary catheter to monitor output
  - cardiac monitoring
  - pulse oximetry
  - regular recording of vital signs
  - warm with hot air blankets
  - warm IV fluids
  - NG tube if there is gastric dilation
  - aim for a rise in temperature of 0.5–1°C per hour
- Rapid warming can cause hypotension and arrhythmias leading to cardiac arrest

:⚙: **Myocardial infarction**

A myocardial infarction (MI) results from an interruption to the blood supply to the myocardium which causes necrosis. It typically presents with central retrosternal pain, which is crushing in nature and may radiate to the jaw, neck, or arms. The patient may collapse due to a sudden reduction in cardiac output. There may be a history of ischaemic heart disease or a family history of cardiac problems. Immediate medical assessment is required.

📖 See Chest pain, p.115.

:⚙: **Poisoning**

Misuse (accidental or deliberate) of many substances can lead to collapse. The commonest presentation is as a result of alcohol ingestion. A full assessment must be undertaken to exclude any underlying pathology or injury.

📖 See Apparently drunk, p.37.

:O: Stroke/transient ischaemic attack

Also referred to as a cerebral vascular event (CVE) or a cerebral vascular accident (CVA), this is the most common neurological disorder and the leading cause of severe disability in the UK. The condition is closely related to transient ischaemic attack (TIA) with the only difference being that a TIA resolves within 24 hours. TIA is an important marker for future stroke with 10% of people who have a TIA going on to have a stroke within the next 12 months and 20% having a stroke at some time in the future. Patients should be referred to a specialist neurovascular clinic within a week of a TIA and admitted to hospital if more than one TIA occurs in a short period of time.

A stroke occurs when the circulation to part of the brain is interrupted resulting in cerebral infarction. There are two main pathologies:

Ischaemia
80% of strokes are caused by an ischaemic event:
- Cerebral thrombosis:
  - atherosclerosis
  - hypertension
- Cerebral embolism:
  - atrial fibrillation
  - post-MI
  - endocarditis
- Hypo-perfusion:
  - cardiac insufficiency
  - haemorrhage
  - severe dehydration

Haemorrhage
The remaining 20% are haemorrhagic events:
- Intracerebral bleed
- Subarachnoid bleed
- Bleeding disorders

Key signs and symptoms
- Depends on the area of the brain affected
- Unilateral neurological signs:
  - weakness—face/limb/slurred speech
  - altered sensation
  - loss of balance
  - visual disturbance
- Headache may be present
- Confusional state
- Collapse

Key history and assessment
- A quick assessment can be undertaken using the FAST mnemonic:
- **F**—Facial weakness:
  - can the patient smile?
  - has their mouth or an eye drooped?

- **A**—Arm weakness:
  - can the patient raise both arms?
- **S**—Speech problems:
  - can the patient speak clearly and understand what you say to them?
- **T**—Test:
  - test all 3 signs
- How long have symptoms been present? If <3 hours consider the possibility of thrombolytic therapy
- Alteration in normal daily activities of living
- Unexplained falls
- History of heart disease particularly atrial fibrillation
- Diabetes
- Hypertension
- Tobacco use
- Alcohol misuse
- Positive family history of stroke or cardiovascular disease

Key observations and findings
- Temperature
- Pulse
- Respiratory rate
- BP
- GCS
- Focal neurological deficit

Key investigations
- Blood glucose
- Urgent CT should be undertaken if the patient has:
  - been taking anticoagulant treatment
  - known bleeding disorder
  - decreased level of consciousness
  - fever
  - severe headache at onset
  - Symptom onset within 3 hours—? thrombolysis
- 12-lead ECG

Key actions and treatment
- Ensure the airway is clear
- High-flow O_2, 15L per min via a non-rebreathing mask
- IV access
- Refer to medical team
- Aspirin 300mg if:
  - patient alert
  - gag reflex is intact
  - haemorrhage has been excluded
- Ensure no injuries are present if patient has fallen
- Attention will be required to pressure area care
- Thrombolytic therapy may be considered within 3 hours of onset of symptoms and haemorrhage has been excluded

ⓘ **Vaso-vagal syncope**

This transient loss of consciousness which results in the patient collapsing and then spontaneously recovering is commonly referred to as fainting. It can occur for a wide varity of reasons in otherwise fit and healthy people.

Triggers include:
- Exposure to prolonged heat
- Intense emotional experience
- Extreme stress
- Pain
- Fear
- Fatigue
- Sudden changes in body position

Whatever the trigger the effect on the body is stimulation of the vagus nerve. This results in a slowing of the heart rate and lowering of the BP. Blood supply to the brain is disrupted and the patient may experience lightheadedness, nausea, hot or cold sweats, visual disturbances, and an awareness that they are going to faint. If he/she cannot lie or sit down then collapse may occur. Once horizontal the blood supply is restored to the brain and the patient quickly regains consciousness. The patient may need to be assessed for injuries resulting from the fall and blood glucose should be checked. If the trigger is identifiable this should be addressed.

Dental problems

Differential diagnosis

:☼: **Urgent presentations**
- Acute swelling of the mouth
- Inhaled tooth
- Ludwig's angina.

① **Timely presentations**
- Avulsed tooth
- Crown fracture
- Dental abscesses
- Minor haemorrhage
- Mucosal infection
- Toothache

⑦ **Non-urgent presentations**
- Ulcers

Introduction

True emergencies affecting the teeth and supporting tissues are uncommon. However, emergency assessment should always include an assessment of the airway, breathing and circulation.

Swelling in the mouth and throat or an inhaled tooth can lead to:
- Airway compromise
- Inadequate breathing

:۞: Acute swelling

Swelling within the mouth is potentially dangerous due to the threat to the airway. Causes include infection and allergic reaction. *Substantial swelling requires urgent experienced medical review.*

📖 See Sore throat, p.391.

:۞: Inhaled tooth

An inhaled tooth may present as a clinical emergency if the tooth is obstructing the airway. *All patients with respiratory distress must be treated as a life-threatening emergency.*

Key signs and symptoms
- Missing tooth
- Coughing
- Respiratory distress

Key history and assessment
- Injury to the jaw/mouth
- Choking sensation

Key observations and findings
- Respiratory rate
- Pulse
- O_2 saturation

Key investigations
- CXR
- ABGs if respiratory distress present

Key actions and treatment
- Urgent referral to experienced clinician for airway management

☼ Ludwig's angina

This is a rapidly progressing, tense bilateral cellulitis of the submandibular, sublingual, and submental spaces. There is gross swelling of the neck and mouth. It is a potential airway emergency with a mortality rate of 75% if not treated rapidly. *Urgent experienced medical review is required.*

📖 See Sore throat, p.391.

! Avulsed tooth

If one or more adult teeth are knocked out, immediate action is required. Delay adversely affects the likelihood of successful re-implantation. First teeth should not be re-implanted, as the developing adult teeth can be damaged in the process.

Key actions and treatment
- The tooth must be kept moist to prevent the cells on the root from drying out
- Handle only by the crown, not the root
- Re-implant adult tooth
- Place tooth in milk if unable to re-implant immediately
- Urgent referral to a dentist

! Crown fractures

Crown fracture can involve any of the following structures:
- Enamel only
- Enamel and dentine
- Enamel, dentine, and pulp
- Crown and root

The possibility that any missing segments may have been inhaled should be considered in all cases.

Key actions and treatment
- All require referral to a dentist
- Provide analgesia

! Dental abscesses

Dental abscesses are extremely painful. Formation of pus occurs under the tooth placing pressure on the nerve.

Key signs and symptoms
- Toothache
- Painful jaw localized to one side
- Pyrexia
- Swelling on the affected side

Key history and assessment
- Increasing pain
- Localized swelling of the jaw

Key observations and findings
- Low grade pyrexia
- Pain score: likely to be severe

Key investigations
- None normally required

Key actions and treatment
- Provide sufficient analgesia
- Advise on ongoing analgesia
- Oral antibiotics according to local guidelines
- Advise to make early appointment with dentist

! Minor haemorrhage

Following injury or surgery to the mouth, bleeding is common and usually appears worse than it is.

Key actions and treatment
- Ensure the airway is not compromised
- Reassure the patient
- Sit the patient upright
- Encourage biting firmly on gauze or dental roll for 20min
- Treat the cause if possible
- Check if the patient is on anticoagulants such as aspirin or warfarin
- May require clotting factors to be checked if bleeding continues
- If unable to control bleeding refer for medical review

① Mucosal infection

>300 different pathogens have been isolated in the human mouth. Good oral hygiene is essential in aiding the antibacterial properties of saliva in ensuring a healthy balance is maintained with the oral cavity. Those unable to maintain a good oral hygiene routine or who are immunocompromised are at greater risk of developing mucosal infection—particularly fungal infection.

Key history and assessment
- Duration and site of pain
- Note location and extent of swelling
- Oral hygiene routine

Key observations
- Check for pyrexia

Key actions and treatment
- Treatment will depend on the causative agent. See local antibiotic guidelines

① Toothache

Whilst not considered a medical emergency, patients often seek emergency treatment due to unremitting pain. It occurs when the dental pulp is inflamed and the only definitive treatment is removal of the pulp.

Key actions and treatment
- Oral analgesia
- Refer to dentist for definitive treatment

⑦ Ulcers

Painful ulcers on the inside of the cheeks, gums, or tongue are very common with the majority of people experiencing them at some time. They can result from trauma such as biting the inside of the mouth, biting finger nails which then damage the mucosa, or vigorous brushing. These ulcers normally heal spontaneously within a week.

Other ulcers may be recurrent, reappearing every few weeks or months. The most common of these are small sores up to 5mm in diameter which may occur singly or in clusters. Rarer are large ulcers which can last for several months or very small herpetiform ulcers which occur in clusters of dozens at a time. Emergency presentation is normally due to pain. Unfortunately regardless of the wide variety of OTC preparations available no one product appears to work consistently for the majority of people.

Key actions and treatment
- Advise patient to try OTC preparations
- If recurrent, refer to primary care physician

Further reading

Perry M (2005). *Head, Neck and Dental Emergencies.* Oxford: Oxford University Press.

Diabetes

Differential diagnosis

☼ **True emergencies**
- Diabetic ketoacidosis
- Hypoglycaemia

Diabetes mellitus

Diabetes mellitus is a chronic metabolic disorder in which the blood glucose becomes too high as a result of cells being unable to access it due to a lack of insulin.

Glucose is normally absorbed from the duodenum after eating. It is also stored in the liver in the form of glycogen. Insulin is released by the pancreas in response to raising levels of blood glucose. It enables the glucose to enter cells where it is further metabolized. Insulin also enables glucose not required immediately by the body to be stored in the liver for future use.

Glucose is the main source of energy for cells and the normal range within the blood stream is between 4–8mmol/L. The brain is most susceptible to acute changes to blood glucose levels.

There are two main types of diabetes—type 1 and type 2.

Type 1
- Insulin-dependent diabetes mellitus (IDDM)
- Younger onset, <40 years old
- Patient unable to produce insulin
- Treatment: insulin injections

Type 2
- Non-insulin-dependent diabetes mellitus (NIDDM)
- More common, up to 95% of all cases
- Strong link to obesity
- Older age of onset
- Insulin is produced but not in sufficient quantities
- Treatment depends on the extent and stage of the problem and may follow a range of treatment including:
  - lifestyle changes such as regular exercise, weight loss, dietary changes
  - oral medication
  - insulin injections

:☠: Diabetic ketoacidosis

DKA is a life-threatening complication of diabetes resulting from a severe deficiency of insulin. In young adults, it may be the first indication that the patient has diabetes. In people with established type 1 diabetes it may occur if their demand for insulin is increased by:

- Infection
- Trauma
- Surgery
- MI

DKA can occur in patients with type 2 diabetes but is less common.

Due to lack of insulin, cells utilize fat as a source of energy. This process produces ketones which alter the blood pH making it acidaemic. Ketones are excreted in urine but increasing blood ketone levels will lead to coma and death if untreated.

Key signs and symptoms

- Polydipsia, excessive thirst
- Polyuria
- Dehydration
- Glycosuria
- Fatigue
- N&V
- Odour of acetone on breath
- Abdominal pain
- Confusion and drowsiness

Key history and assessment

- History of vomiting, drowsiness, and increased confusion over 2–3 days
- History of polyuria and polydipsia
- Concurrent infection
- Poorly controlled or poorly managed diabetes

Key observations and findings

- Raised blood glucose level >15mmol/L
- Kussmaul's breathing: deep sighing characteristic
- Ketones on breath and in the urine
- Electrolyte imbalance (hyperkalaemia) may be noted on ABG

Key investigations

- ABGs
- U&Es
- FBC
- ECG
- Cardiac enzymes
- CXR if chest infection suspected
- Blood, urine, and sputum for culture if indicated

Key actions and observations

- Maintain airway if necessary
- Rehydration with isotonic IV fluids

- Monitor blood glucose levels
- Monitor urinary output, catheterize if necessary
- Insulin infusion according to local guidelines
- Regular vital signs monitoring
- ECG monitoring
- NG tube if conscious level is impaired
- Refer to in patient medical team

☠ Hypoglycaemia

Hypoglycaemia is the most common emergency presentation in diabetics and is most commonly seen in patients with type 1 diabetes. It occurs when blood glucose levels fall too low, normally as a result of:

- Too much insulin
- Missed meal resulting in insufficient glucose
- Too much oral medication
- High utilization of glucose due to exercise

Blood glucose must always be measured in patients presenting with:

- Seizures
- Abnormal behaviour
- Apparent alcohol intoxication

Key signs and symptoms

- Sweating
- Pallor
- Hunger
- Irritability and confusion
- Atypical behaviour
- Lethargy
- Loss of coordination
- Tremor
- Visual disturbance
- Unconsciousness
- Seizures: glucose must be checked in patients presenting with a seizure

Key history and assessment

- Known IDDM
- History of missed meals
- History of recent illness e.g. diarrhoea and vomiting

Key observations and findings

- Reduced conscious level: record GCS
- Low blood glucose level: <3.5mmol/L

Key investigations

- Check blood glucose

Key actions and treatment

- Maintain airway and ensure adequate breathing if necessary
- If conscious: give fast acting glucose drink or gel
- If unconscious:
  - 50mL 50% glucose IV—into a large vein as this solution is an irritant
  - glucagon 1mg by IM injection
  - may require an IV glucose infusion
- Check blood glucose after 15–20min
- If the cause has been identified, and patient can be accompanied home, may be able to discharge
- May require referral to:
  - inpatient team
  - outpatient follow-up appointment

- diabetic specialist nurse
- Primary Care
- May require admission if:
  - Blood glucose difficult to control
  - Concurrent illness
  - Patient on oral hypoglycaemics—as hypoglycaemia will recur

Diarrhoea and vomiting

Differential diagnosis

☼ **Urgent presentations**
- Dehydration
- Haematemesis
- Rectal bleeding

① **Timely assessment**
- Gastroenteritis

Introduction

Diarrhoea and vomiting (D&V) are common symptoms of a wide range of pathology. They can occur alone or together. Current and recent drug therapy (particularly antibiotics) should be considered along with the potential for environmental exposure to infection. In the majority of cases D&V is a minor illness. However, if the condition is prolonged underlying pathology should be investigated and excluded. Most emergency presentations occur due to the severity of the symptoms, the inconvenience caused to the patient, or the sudden onset.

Diarrhoea

Diarrhoea may be acute or chronic and is defined as the passing of loose stools. The condition is usually infective in origin resulting from inflammation of the bowel. Important considerations involve the severity of the diarrhoea, presence of blood, coexisting medical conditions and the age of the patient (i.e. very young or elderly). In most cases diarrhoea resolves within a week.

Causes
- Infection
- Excessive laxative use
- Food intolerance or allergy
- Drugs e.g. antibiotics
- Constipation with overflow
- Irritable bowel syndrome
- GI bleed
- Diverticular disease
- Bowel obstruction
- Coeliac disease
- Inflammatory bowel disease
- Tumour

Vomiting

Vomiting is most commonly infective in origin. Prolonged vomiting, high grade pyrexia or haematemesis requires investigation. Excessive vomiting can lead to dehydration which may require admission for IV fluids. Patients who are vomiting should have their airway checked to ensure it is clear. This is particularly important in those with an altered conscious level who may have a reduced or absent gag reflex and therefore are unable to protect their airway.

Causes
- Infection
- Alcohol excess
- Motion sickness/labyrinthitis
- MI
- Small bowel obstruction
- Trauma: head/abdomen
- Pregnancy
- Eating disorders: self-induced

☼ Dehydration

Dehydration may occur when fluid loss exceeds the patient's intake. The risk is greater where the patient has a fever and in those with pre-existing medical problems such as diabetes.

Indicators of dehydration

- Dry mouth, tongue, or lips
- Reduced skin turgor
- Sunken eyes
- Thirst
- Headache
- Light-headedness
- Tiredness
- Confusion and irritability
- Reduced urine output
- Concentrated urine
- Hypotension
- Tachycardia
- Tachypnoea

Dehydration may be mild, moderate, or severe. Mild or moderate cases may be treated by giving the patient frequent sips of clear fluids or commercially available oral rehydration solutions. If the dehydration is more severe then IV rehydration may be required. In more severe cases U&Es should be checked and abnormalities corrected. In extreme cases hypovolaemic shock may occur which requires urgent and aggressive intervention.

✪ Haematemesis

The presence of any blood in the vomit should give rise to concern and prompt immediate medical review. The type of bleeding and quantity should be noted. This can range from a small number of red flecks of blood to the vomiting of large quantities of fresh blood. The latter is a clinical emergency and requires immediate IV access, fluids, and senior medical assessment. The vomiting of dark, granular, coffee-ground vomit may indicate the presence of partially digested blood in the stomach.

Potential causes
- Peptic ulceration
- Acute gastritis
- Mallory–Weiss tear
- Oesophageal varices
- Epistaxis—vomiting of ingested blood
- Ingestion of corrosive substance
- Ruptured oesophagus

✪ Rectal bleeding

Rectal bleeding can occur from the colon, rectum, or anus. The majority of episodes are mild and self-limiting and resolve without treatment. The patient may notice a few drops of blood when wiping themselves. Other patients may report passing clots along with stool. In more severe cases, large quantities of fresh blood may be passed and the patient is at risk of developing hypovolaemia. Treatment depends upon the severity of bleeding and can range from advice about diet and avoiding constipation to intravenous fluid resuscitation.

Causes
- Haemorrhoids
- Anal fissure
- Diverticulosis
- Infection
- Colitis
- Neoplasm

The passage of melaena—black, tarry, offensive-smelling stools—indicates bleeding from the upper GI tract, normally as a result of peptic ulceration.

ⓘ **Gastroenteritis**

Gastroenteritis is the most common cause for D&V, affecting 20% of the population in the UK each year. It is normally treated at home without medical intervention.

Key signs and symptoms

- Loose stools
- Vomiting of stomach contents:
  - usually contains partially digested food
  - may be bile stained
- Loss of appetite
- Abdominal cramps
- Malaise
- Signs of dehydration

Key history and assessment

- Check onset, duration, and frequency of symptoms
- History of recent travel
- Recent food intake
- Assess type of diarrhoea and vomit
- Any medications taken, including OTC drugs
- Any affected contacts
- Occupation, especially relevant if the patient is a food handler or healthcare worker
- Assess for signs of dehydration

Key observations and findings

- Check temperature
- Pulse: may be raised if dehydrated
- Respiration: may be raised if dehydrated
- BP: should be normal

Key investigations

- Blood tests are not usually required unless significant dehydration present
- U&Es: may demonstrate severity of electrolyte abnormalities
- Stool cultures: to isolate infective agent
- Blood cultures: if systemic infection suspected

Key actions and treatment

- Ensure patient is able to protect their own airway
- Rehydrate with oral fluids if tolerated
- Increase oral fluid intake gradually using clear fluids or rehydration sachets
- Give mouth care after each vomiting episode
- In severe vomiting, IV fluids may be needed to rehydrate
- Consider the use of anti-emetics
- Maintain good standards of hygiene to prevent spread
- Some types of food poisoning are notifiable in the UK

Ear problems

Differential diagnosis

① **Timely assessment**

- Wounds

② **Non-urgent presentations**

- Barotrauma
- Cholesteatoma
- Foreign bodies
- Hair follicle infection in the ear canal
- Otitis externa
- Otitis media
- Ruptured eardrum
- Vertigo

Introduction

Problems with the ears are unlikely to require emergency or urgent intervention. Most emergency presentations are due to the pain and discomfort which occurs with a number of ear conditions. Effective management of pain can allow the patient to be further assessed or referred on as appropriate. Pain may also be referred from dental conditions, the temporo-mandibular joint, tonsillitis, pharyngitis, or neck problems.

⊙ Wounds

Wounds to the ear are common and occur often during contact sports or as the result of an assault. They require careful assessment and management to ensure a good cosmetic result.

Key signs and symptoms
- Obvious wound to the pinna or lobe

Key history and assessment
- Mechanism of injury
- Exclude the possibility of a human bite
- Assess injury to the cartilage
- Assess for skin loss

Key observations and findings
- None normally required

Key investigations
- None normally required

Key actions and treatment
- Simple skin wounds may be closed by application of adhesive strips or glue
- Involvement of the cartilage or the pinna requires medical review
- Risk of infection following a bite is high, through cleaning and medical review is required

⑦ Barotrauma

Barotrauma is the presence of pain or discomfort in the ear as a result of sudden changes to the pressure within the middle ear. The air pressure in the middle ear is normally atmospheric. This is maintained by the Eustachian tube. If the tube is not patent then the difference between the pressure in the middle ear and the atmosphere cannot be equalized. This causes pain as the tympanic membrane is strained. The commonest cause is URTI.

It can occur during any event which results in pressure changes, e.g., air travel or diving. The majority of cases are resolved by the patient themselves (e.g. yawning, sucking on sweets). If these actions fail then health care may be sought. The problem should resolve without intervention.

Key signs and symptoms
- Pain may be unilateral or bilateral
- Pain can range from mild discomfort to severe pain
- Reduction in hearing
- Feeling of congestion in the ear

Key history and assessment
- History of sudden onset of signs and symptoms
- Recent exposure to pressure changes
- Bulging or retraction of the eardrum

Key observations and findings
- None normally required

Key investigations
- None required

Key actions and treatment
- Advice on actions to assist equalization of pressure
- Advice on preventive actions for future occasions

⑦ Cholesteatoma

This condition occurs in the middle ear most commonly following a problem with the Eustachian tube. If the tube does not close properly negative pressure occurs, pulling the rear of the tympanic membrane backwards. Sometimes perforation of the eardrum following trauma or chronic infection can cause excessive skin growth from the outer side of the eardrum into the middle ear. Either event results in the development of a cyst which sheds skin cells as it grows. The accumulation of the dead cells form a focus for further infection and the production of enzymes which erode the adjoining bones and can, in the worse case, cause intracranial infection.

Key signs and symptoms
- Intermittent drainage from the ear, which may be offensive
- Feeling of pressure within the ear
- Reduction in hearing
- Discomfort behind the ear, worse when lying down

Key history and assessment
- Granulation tissue may be seen on examination of the tympanic membrane
- The build up of dead cells may be seen as white debris within the ear

Key observations and findings
- Temperature should be taken to assess the extent of the infection

Key investigations
- None required prior to referral

Key actions and treatment
- Requires referral to ENT for further assessment

⑦ Foreign bodies

FBs in the external ear canal are a relatively common presentation. These are usually placed in the ear in an attempt to remove wax. Insects may also fly into the ear and be unable to get out. Ear piercings can migrate into the lobe or work themselves under the skin covering the cartilage.

📖 See Foreign bodies, p.233.

⑦ Hair follicle infection in the ear canal

An infection in a hair follicle within the ear canal results in a small abscess. The causative agent is usually *Staphylococcus aureus*.

Key signs and symptoms
- Severe pain in the ear canal, increasing if the ear is touched or moved
- Unilateral reduction in hearing

Key history and assessment
- History of pain in the ear increasing over a few days
- Inflammation of the ear canal

Key observations and findings
- Check temperature to ensure the patient is not pyrexial

Key investigations
- None required

Key actions and treatment
- Analgesia
- Antibiotics
- Will require follow-up in Primary Care if the infection does not settle within a few days

⑦ Otitis externa

Inflammation of the external ear canal occurs in response to infection, an allergen or an irritant such as shampoo, or recurrent dampness. It is more common in swimmers and after minor trauma, such as that caused by inserting objects into the ear to remove wax.

Key signs and symptoms
- Unilateral inflamed external ear canal

Key history and assessment
- Pain on palpation of the tragus or pinna

Key observations and findings
- Temperature, pulse, and respiratory rate

Key investigations
- None required

Key actions and treatment
- Antibiotic and anti-inflammatory ear drops
- Paracetamol or NSAIDs for pain
- Avoid causative actions if identifiable
- ENT referral if tympanic membrane is not visible

⑦ Otitis media

Although more common in children, infection of the middle ear can also occur in adults. The build up of mucus behind the tympanic membrane causes increased pressure resulting in pain. The condition usually resolves within 72 hours. Management is primarily aimed at pain relief. Occasionally the pressure causes the tympanic membrane to perforate resulting in purulent discharge and some relief of pain. The perforation heals within a few weeks.

Key signs and symptoms
- Severe earache
- Pyrexia
- Hearing reduction
- Severe cases may cause vomiting

Key history and assessment
- History of recent or current URTI
- Inflamed, bulging tympanic membrane
- Loss of light reflex from tympanic membrane
- Check the mastoid process for pain, redness, and swelling which may indicate mastoiditis. This is rare but serious and can result in bone necrosis and intracranial infection. If suspected urgent ENT referral is required

Key observations and findings
- Temperature, pulse, and respiratory rate

Key investigations
- None required

Key actions and treatment
- Analgesia as required to manage pain and antipyretics for the fever. Paracetamol or NSAIDs are often suitable
- There is no evidence that antibiotics have any effect on the course of the infection
- Follow-up in Primary Care for recurrent episodes

⑦ Ruptured eardrum

Perforation of the tympanic membrane may occur following trauma or infection. Direct blows to the ear during sport or an assault, blast injuries, and basal skull fractures can all cause ruptures. Attempts to clean ears with a cotton bud may also result in a perforation.

Key signs and symptoms
- Pain accompanies the rupture but then subsides, especially if it occurs as part of an infection
- Reduction in hearing
- Tinnitus may be present if the rupture was the result of a severe blow or large explosion

Key history and assessment
- History of traumatic event
- History of ear infection
- Perforation visible on examination

Key observations and findings
- None normally required

Key investigations
- None normally required

Key actions and treatment
- Advise that most heal spontaneously
- Advise to keep the ear dry, avoid swimming
- ENT follow-up to ensure healing

⑦ Vertigo

The sensation of movement while stationary can range from a barely perceptible sensation through to an inability to stand or the feeling that a room is spinning while lying down. Mild attacks are common and are usually the result of viral labyrinthitis, resolving without treatment. A number of other illnesses can also cause the condition. These all require further investigation:

- Benign positional vertigo
- Meniérè's disease
- Vestibular neuronitis
- Chronic otitis media
- Acoustic neuroma
- Cholesteatoma
- Stroke
- Head injury
- Multiple sclerosis

Key signs and symptoms
- Sensation of movement while still
- Sensation of light-headedness, often described as feeling slightly drunk or vomiting
- Associated signs of ear infection

Key history and assessment
- Type of onset: sudden or gradual?
- Previous episodes: if so, how long did they last?
- Drug history
- History of a recent head injury

Key observations and findings
- Temperature, pulse, respiratory rate, and BP

Key investigations
- None normally required

Key actions and treatment
- Other conditions which may cause light-headedness or dizziness must be excluded. These include anything which may result in hypoxia
- Treatment will be based on the severity of the symptoms
- Mild cases can be referred to primary care, severe causes will require ENT assessment

Exposure to chemicals

Differential diagnosis

Emergency presentations
- Inhalation injury
- Chemical eye injury

Urgent presentations
- Chemical burns

Introduction

Patients exposed to toxic chemicals present very difficult management issues for healthcare professionals. The first principle when dealing with people exposed to chemicals is that they must be decontaminated prior to medical intervention. *It is extremely important to ensure that the carer does not become contaminated.*

Contingency plans for management of exposure should be developed for all services to which the public has access. Fire and Rescue Services and local industries which use potentially hazardous chemicals should be involved in the development of these plans.

In areas which are equipped to deal with contaminated patients regular training will help to ensure that staff are competent to deal with incidents should they arise. In the UK, County Emergency Planning Officers are available to advise on the management of chemical exposures and decontamination procedures. Any company using chemicals which may be considered potentially harmful have to comply with the COSHH Regulations 2002. Companies should hold COSHH datasheets which provide advice regarding health risks and the treatment which may be required should someone be exposed to toxic substances. Information may also be obtained from Toxbase (National Poisons Information Service) which is available free to registered users within the UK National Health Service.

Staff dealing with patients exposed to chemicals should have access to and be trained in the use of personal protective equipment (PPE). They should be familiar with the principles of decontamination and understand the limitations of care which can be given whilst wearing PPE.

:☠: Inhalation injury

Chemical inhalation injury is often associated with combustion and therefore may be combined with the effects of heat damage to the lungs and airway. CO inhalation may occur as a result of the inhalation of car exhaust fumes either accidentally, or as a result of a suicide attempt, or due to faulty combustion from gas appliances. Other inhalation injuries may result from industrial processes if there is inadequate ventilation. When dealing with victims of chemical inhalation it is important to realise that what they are exhaling may also be toxic, and therefore measures should be taken to protect staff from inhaling these fumes and becoming victims themselves.

The airway and lungs are at particular risk in these patients. Assessment and treatment should follow the principles of airway, breathing, and circulation. All patients should be assessed urgently by an experienced doctor.

📖 See Overdose and poisoning, p.313.

☠ Chemical eye injury

Chemical injuries to the eye are a common presentation as a result of contamination by household or industrial chemicals. The patient presents with a history of chemical injury and a painful, red watering eye. It is essential to identify the chemical involved. Alkalis, which raise the pH above 8, cause the most damage as they penetrate through corneal tissue causing extensive intra-ocular damage. Acids lower the pH below 7 and cause localized damage but do not normally penetrate.

Immediate irrigation of the eye with normal saline until the pH returns to normal is required. A high flow rate of saline via an IV giving set is effective. If available, an irrigation lens can be used.

📖 See Eye problems, p.183.

☤ Chemical burns

Chemical burns pose particular problems as tissue damage can continue until the substance is completely removed or neutralized. Alkalis have greater potential to cause serious tissue damage as they continue to penetrate whereas acids cause proteins to coagulate, limiting the degree of tissue penetration.

Irrigation is the main treatment and should be commenced as soon as possible. It is important to consider that some chemical burns can be complicated by systemic absorption of the substance involved.

📖 See Burns and scalds, p.97.

Eye problems

Differential diagnosis

☺ True emergencies
- Acute glaucoma
- Chemical injury

☼ Urgent presentations
- Blunt trauma
- Penetrating eye injury

① Timely assessment
- Arc eye
- Detached retina
- Foreign body
- Keratitis
- Uveitis

⑦ Non-urgent presentations
- Blepharitis
- Conjunctivitis
- Hordeolum stye
- Subconjunctival haemorrhage

Introduction

Acute eye problems are a common emergency presentation. An accurate history of the problems must be ascertained and should include:

- Activity when the symptoms commenced
- Length of time since the onset of symptoms
- Rapidity of onset
- Current status of symptoms
- Severity of pain
- Type of pain
- Visual changes and disturbances
- Presence of discharge
- Photophobia
- N&V
- Normal visual status if known to patient
- Past medical history, including visual health
- Any concurrent medical problems

The visual acuity of both eyes should be tested and recorded in all patients. Using a Snellen chart (Fig. 18.1) each eye is tested independently, with the other eye covered. The patient starts reading the letters on the chart commencing with the largest at the top and working their way down until unable to clearly identify a letter. It may be necessary to instill local anaesthetic (LA) drops to enable the patient to undertake this test. Amethocaine 1% or oxybuprocaine 0.4% are commonly used. If a patient normally wears glasses these should be used where possible. This should be recorded in the patient's history.

Visual acuity should be recorded as a fraction in relation to the last line of the chart read by the patient. Normal vision is considered to be 6/6. If the patient can only read at 6m what a person with normal eyesight would read at 36m than acuity would be recorded as 6/36. Where the patient does not complete a line then it may be recorded by counting the number of letters on the line read accurately (for example 6/9+2 or 6/12+3).

If visual acuity is <6/9 a pinhole card may be used to reduce refractive error. The results with and without the use of a pinhole should be recorded. If the patient is unable to see even the largest letters then the distance to the chart should be shortened by half and this recorded. For example, if the distance to the chart is halved then the recording would be 3/last line read. If the patient cannot see a letter at 1m then the ability to count fingers at 1m should be recorded. If this is absent, perception of hand movement should be tested and if this fails then perception to light is tested.

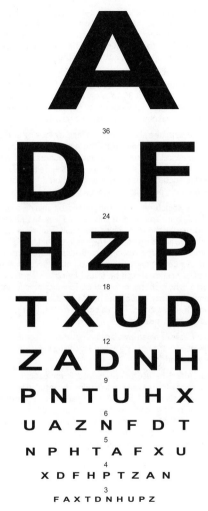

Fig. 18.1 A Snellen chart

Visual fields can be assessed using a confrontation test. The patient is placed 0.5m from the tester and covers one eye, looking straight ahead at the tester with the other. The tester places his/her hand between the patient and themselves to determine whether the patient can see the number of fingers held up in each quadrant of the peripheral vision.

Extraocular muscle function can be tested using a corneal light reflex, the Hirschberg test. With the patient looking straight ahead a light is shone towards their eye from about 30cm away. The light should fall on exactly the same spot on the corneas of both eyes. Asymmetry suggests deviation in alignment due to eye muscle weakness or paralysis.

The external eye structure should be examined by looking at the external points and gradually working inwards. The eyebrows, eyelids, and lashes should be symmetrical. There should be no redness or swelling. Eyes should not protrude or have a sunken appearance. Relaxed facial expressions accompany adequate vision. Lower lids should have blood vessels visible. The eye should be moist and glossy.

The anterior eye structures can be inspected by shining a light on the cornea and checking for smoothness and clarity. There should be no cloudiness of the cornea or the lens behind the pupil. The iris is normally flat with a regular shape and even colour. The pupils should be equal and react to light. When checking the response to light the torch should be held in front of the eye before switching it on to help detect small responses. The cross pupillary reflex should be tested by observing the reaction of one eye when a light is shone in the other. This indicates an intact visual pathway. Examination may include the need to instill fluorescein drops, an orange dye which shows green when a blue (Wood's) light is shone on to it in the presence of corneal damage.

The fundus can be examined by using an ophthalmoscope, although the pupil normally needs dilating using a mydriatic drug in order for structures to be clearly visualized.

The only reason for the use of an eye pad is for patient comfort. It is deemed unnecessary to pad the eye following the instillation of LA due to the short period of time it is effective. If the patient feels it is of no benefit then it should be not be used. If the eye is to be padded then a first pad should be folded in half horizontally and placed into the orbit, a second pad should be placed on top of this and held in place by tape. The patient should be warned that their ability to judge distances will be affected and under no circumstances should they drive with an eye pad in situ. If both eyes are affected by a condition, the worse eye should be padded if the patient wishes.

☠ Acute glaucoma

Sudden blockage of the drainage mechanism for the aqueous humour from the anterior chamber through the canal of Schlemm causes raised intraocular pressure. The resulting constriction of the blood flow to the optic nerve can result in blindness.

Key signs and symptoms

- Sudden onset of symptoms
- Severe pain radiating through the eye affecting the whole head
- N&V
- Pain worse in dimmed light
- Visual defect include blurred vision, and the presence of halos around lights
- Fixed, semi-dilated, oval-shaped pupil

Key history and assessment

- Patient aged >40 years
- History of long sightedness
- Inspect external eye structure
- Inspect anterior eye structures: anterior chamber may be seen to be bulging

Key observations and findings

- Baseline TPR and BP observations
- Check pupils for size, equality, and reaction: the pupil will be fixed and dilated
- Test visual acuity if possible

Key actions and treatments

- *Immediate referral to an ophthalmologist*: early treatment is vital if the eyesight is to be preserved
- Oral or IV analgesia
- Anti-emetics
- The miotic drug pilocarpine 2% as an eye drop every 5min can be used to constrict the pupil. This allows the angle towards the canal to be opened improving drainage of the aqueous humour and therefore reducing pressure build-up
- IV cannula required
- IV fluids may be needed if the patient is dehydrated due to vomiting

☠ Chemical injury

Chemical injuries commonly occur as a result of acidic or alkaline solutions being splashed in the eye. They require immediate first aid and attention. Despite any treatment already given, irrigation should commence at once.

Key signs and symptoms
- Painful eye
- Extreme watering of the eye
- Reluctance to open eye
- Agitated patient due to pain and discomfort
- Vision impairment
- Photophobia

Key history and assessment
- Do not delay treatment by obtaining history
- Chemical involved
- Mechanism of injury
- Normal vision for the patient
- Use of glasses or lenses
- Contact lenses in situ
- Assess visual acuity once irrigation completed
- Examine for corneal erosion using fluorescein
- Assess for any other injury

Key observations and findings
- None required immediately

Key investigations
- None initially

Key actions and treatments
- Minimizing the contact time of the chemical is vital in limiting the amount of damage done
- Remove contact lenses if present
- Remove visible foreign material such as cement
- Copious amounts of normal saline should be irrigated across the affected eye via an IV giving set or an irrigation lens until the pH returns to normal
- The use of LA may be necessary to relieve pain and allow the eye to be opened sufficiently in order to allow irrigation
- Refer all chemical injuries to an ophthalmologist for ongoing treatment and follow-up

☼ Blunt trauma

Blunt trauma to the eye and the surrounding orbit is a common event. It may occur as a result of assault, sporting injury, etc. Small objects which can fit within the orbit, such as squash balls or golf balls, cause the most damage. Eye trauma may also occur in combination with other major injuries.

Key signs and symptoms

- Black eye—ecchymosis
- Hyphaema—bleeding into the anterior chamber, visible as a fluid level in front of the iris
- Fixed dilated pupil—traumatic mydriasis
- Dislocation or subluxation of the lens
- Irregular pupil

Key history and assessment

- History of the incident needs to be fully ascertained
- The eyelids must be opened to facilitate examination of the eye. This can be difficult in the presence of oedema and gross swelling
- Associated injuries should be identified and treated—particularly head and cervical spine injuries

Key observations and findings

- Vital signs should be assessed and recorded
- Visual acuity should be assessed
- Level of consciousness must be assessed to exclude head injury

Key investigations

- Facial and orbital XRs may be required following discussion with an experienced clinician

Key actions and treatments

- Undertake primary survey in line with major trauma guidelines
- Specific treatment will depend on the injuries present
- Refer to ophthalmologist for full assessment
- If a hyphaema is present the patient should be kept sitting upright if possible to allow bleeding to settle

:⚙: Penetrating eye injury

In small penetrating wounds a prolapsing iris may seal the leak. Major penetrating injuries are obvious and can cause fear and panic in patients who often believe they will lose vision permanently in the affected eye. Common incidents occur while gardening, with canes or branches injuring eyes; during assaults especially if glass is involved; or as a result of thrown objects. Smaller particles may also penetrate the eye, for example pieces of metal thrown off while hammering or chiselling or other material projected by power tools. Small injuries may be overlooked or dismissed as superficial FBs. Depending on the mechanism of injury damage may also occur to the eyelid or the soft tissue surrounding the orbit. Head injuries may also need to be excluded.

Key signs and symptoms
- Obvious penetrating trauma
- Visual disturbance
- Pain in the eye
- Distortion of the pupil or iris
- Redness and swelling to the eye or surrounding area
- Watery discharging eye, aqueous fluid, blood, or tearing
- Headache as a result of direct eye trauma

Key history and assessment
- Mechanism of injury
- Use of protective eyewear
- Exposure to the risk of high velocity particles
- Decreased visual acuity
- Headache
- Decreased level of consciousness—significant head injury
- Check visual acuity
- Check pupils for size, equality, and reaction against observational chart
- Inspect external eye structure
- Test visual fields
- Past medical history

Key observations and findings
- Assess vital signs: should be normal, although may be tachycardic, tachypnoea, or hypertensive due to pain and/or anxiety
- Regular neurological observations, every 15min if any indication of an accompanying head injury

Key investigations
- Plain XR, orbital XR, or ultrasound may be required.
- CT scans may be required
- If injury is likely to require surgical intervention then:
  - FBC, U&Es as baselines
  - cross-match, group and save
  - blood glucose level

Key actions and treatments

- *DO NOT attempt to remove FB*
- Immediate referral to ophthalmologist
- Protect any retained FBs with a gallipot if possible
- Place sterile pad lightly over eye for protection
- Keep head as still as possible to minimize any further damage
- Antibiotics may be recommended by ophthalmologist
- Protect patient from injury due to disorientation and cognitive impaired function, use of cot sides, pillows etc.
- Assess patient for any associated injuries
- Analgesia for pain

! Arc eye

Also known as welders' flash or snow blindness. It is caused by exposure to ultra violet light without wearing adequate eye protection. It results in an acute and superficial keratitis with inflammation seen as redness surrounding the cornea.

Key signs and symptoms
- Usually bilateral
- Inflammation may be seen surrounding the cornea
- Pain: usually severe
- Photophobia
- Inability to open eye due to pain
- FB sensation
- Watery eyes
- The eyelid may have muscular spasms: blepharospasm

Key history and assessment
- How long have symptoms been present?
- History of exposure to UV light, welding, sunbed use, skiing
- Decreased visual acuity
- Watering eyes
- Severity of pain
- Photophobia
- The cornea should be examined carefully for signs of abrasions or ulcers under the blue light on a slit lamp. LA may be required for this
- Staining the eye with fluorescein and observation with a slit lamp will be necessary to identify any superficial particles or corneal erosion

Key observations and findings
- Visual acuity must be recorded

Key investigation
- None required

Key actions and treatment
- Oral analgesia if required
- The eye may be patched for patient comfort
- Mydriatics (e.g. cyclopentolate) to relieve ciliary spasm and pain
- LA drops must not be given to the patient for regular use as they delay the healing
- Refer to ophthalmologist if no improvement within 48 hours

! Detached retina

Detachment of the retina from the choroid as a result of trauma, diabetes, or idiopathic in the elderly. It can also follow cataract surgery.

Key signs and symptoms
- Patient complains of flashing lights—tearing of the retina
- Loss of vision
- Complete loss of vision may occur if left untreated
- Usually painless

Key history and assessment
- Middle aged or older
- Nearsightedness
- Previous cataract surgery
- Glaucoma
- Diabetes
- Trauma
- Previous retinal detachment
- Family history of retinal detachment

Key observations and findings
- Visual acuity reduced

Key actions and treatments
- Refer to ophthalmology

! **Foreign bodies**

FBs in the eye are a common problem. Often they are small pieces of dirt, dust, grit, or plant material blown into the eye by the wind. They can also be wood or metal particles thrown in during a work process or insects which fly into the eye. Most often they are conjunctival and are washed by the lacrimal process into the lower fornix. They may be sub tarsal becoming fixed under the upper lid or they may be corneal, becoming embedded into the cornea. Discomfort is usually out of proportion to the size of the FB. On occasion the FB itself may have been removed from the eye by watering or by the patient wiping it, but the patient still feels that it is in situ. This can be as a result of a corneal abrasion being present caused by the FB scratching the surface of the cornea. Corneal abrasions may also be caused by objects such as fingernails.

Key signs and symptoms
- FB sensation
- Pain
- Excessive watering
- Inability to open eye due to discomfort
- Photophobia

Key history and assessment
- May or may not be a history of FB entering the eye
- History of exposure to dusty or windy environment

Key observations and findings
- Reduce visual acuity due to excessive watering

Key actions and treatment
- Instill LA drops to facilitate examination and removal of FB
- Thorough examination of the eye, including eversion of both lids
- Remove any visible FB with a moist cotton bud
- Embedded corneal FB may be removed by a competent practitioner using the side edge of a 21G needle
- After removal the eye should be stained with fluorescein to assess for corneal abrasions
- Ophthalmology follow-up should be considered if not all of the FB was removed or a rust ring from metal is present

ⓘ **Keratitis**

Keratitis is a general term for a number of conditions which result in inflammation of the cornea and subsequent necrosis and ulceration. The condition can occur following an abrasion caused by a FB or an injury. It may also be infective in origin; herpes simplex is the most serious infection as it may result in permanent loss of vision. Keratitis may also be due to the surface of the cornea becoming dry and ulcerated as a result of insufficient closing of the eyelid, prolonged opening of the eye lid in unconscious patients, inadequate tear production, prolonged contact lens wearing, or exposure to intense ultraviolet light sources such as snow blindness or welding. Systemic disorders, particularly autoimmune conditions or vitamin A deficiency, may also cause keratitis.

Key signs and symptoms
- Pain
- Photophobia
- FB sensation
- Inflammation may be seen as redness surrounding the cornea
- Visual disturbance
- Watering eyes
- The eyelid may have muscular spasms—blepharospasm

Key history and assessment
- How long have symptoms been present?
- Any visual disturbances?
- Inspect intraocular muscle function
- Inspect external eye structure
- Inspect anterior structures
- Observe the anterior chamber: there may be pus present—hypopyon
- The patient complaining of feeling systemically unwell

Key observations and findings
- Check pupils for size, equality, and reaction
- Test visual acuity
- Test visual fields

Key actions and treatments
- No treatment should be given as the condition requires referral to ophthalmologist
- Correct identification of the cause is vital: suspected herpes simplex infection is an ophthalmological emergency
- Discontinue use of contact lenses until infection clears
- Possible complications include, ulceration of the cornea, glaucoma, permanent scarring, and loss of vision

⏀ Uveitis

Inflammation of the uveal tract, which consists of the iris, choroids, and ciliary muscles. Anterior uveitis, or iritis, is inflammation of the iris; inflammation of the ciliary body is known as iridocyclitis; posterior uveitis is choroiditis; and when anterior and posterior is combined it is referred to as pan-uveitis. Uveitis is often idiopathic but can be the result of trauma or systemic conditions as ulcerative colitis, ankylosing spondylitis, or rheumatoid disease.

Key signs and symptoms
- Pain
- Blurring of vision and presence of floaters
- Photophobia
- The iris may go into spasms and cause a constricted pupil
- Pupil may be irregular due to adhesions—synechiae
- Hazy cornea
- Circumcorneal injection

Key history and assessment
- Observe for the presence of pus in the anterior chamber—hypopyon
- Inspect anterior eye structures
- Pain increases on convergence and accommodation of pupils
- Pain in affected eye if a light is shone in the other eye
- Past medical history for related conditions

Key observations and findings
- Pupils for size, equality, and reaction
- Test visual acuity

Key investigations
- None normally required until assessed by an ophthalmologist.

Key actions and treatments
- Urgent referral to an ophthalmologist

⑦ Blepharitis

Inflammation of the eyelid which may be generalized or localized and is often worse at the lid margins. It is a chronic condition in which acute episodes occur.

Key signs and symptoms
- Eye irritation/dry eye sensation
- Burning sensation
- Watering and tearing
- FB sensation
- Crusty debris within the lashes
- Redness of the eyelid margins

Key actions and treatments
- Refer to ophthalmologist
- Advice on bathing the eyelid, ensuring removal of all discharge
- Topical antibiotics

⑦ Conjunctivitis

Inflammation of the conjunctiva is one of the most common eye disorders. It is often allergic in response to pollen, animal hair, or other local allergen. In adults it is usually viral, often secondary or other infections such as the common cold. If bacterial, *Staphylococcus, Pneumococcus,* can be causative agents. Conjunctivitis in infants <2 months is an ophthalmological emergency and requires immediate referral.

Key signs and symptoms
- Injected redness of the conjunctiva
- Gritty sensation in the eye
- Feelings of discomfort in the eye
- Viral: may be unilateral but often bilateral, itchy, watery, patient complains eye feels dry despite the watering, follicular swelling present on everting lid, may feel unwell due to other factors like common cold symptoms
- Bacterial: may be unilateral but often bilateral, sticky eyelids, worse first thing in the morning, the eye may become stuck/closed due to discharge
- Allergic: bilateral, swelling of the eyelids, puffy eyes, irritation in the eyes, not normally painful

Key history and assessment
- When was the onset?
- Any visual problems or decreased acuity?
- Any pain?
- Recent cold or other infections?
- Any discharge? If present then type, quantity, colour. Is the discharge purulent and yellow?
- Do crusts form at night?
- Any previous allergies?
- Exposure to new substances, makeup, contact lens solution, animals, cleaning products, pollen?
- Any family members or other contacts with a similar condition?

Key observations and findings
- None normally required
- May be mild pyrexia and tachycardia if other infection present

Key investigations
- None required

Key actions and treatments
- Allergic: self-limiting, remove allergen from patient or patient from allergen, systemic antihistamines may be helpful
- Viral: artificial tears may help with dry eyes. Infection with adenovirus is highly contagious. Extreme care needs to be taken with hand washing and ensuring towels, face clothes etc. are washed frequently and not shared in order to prevent the spread of infection
- Bacterial: antibacterial cream or drops such as chloramphenicol or sodium fusidate (Fucidin®)

- Warm water to bath crusted eye to encourage opening
- Swabs should be used in one direction when bathing the eye, from the midline outwards
- Treat as infectious by direct and indirect contact. Strict hand washing before and after application of treatment. Towels etc. should only be used by infected party and not the rest of the family
- Refer to ophthalmologist if not improving after 24 hours

⑦ Episcleritis

The episclera is a transparent layer which sits between the sclera and the conjunctiva. The cause for its inflammation is normally unknown, although it is thought people suffering from arthritis experience higher incidences than the general population.

Key signs and symptoms
- Unilateral
- Defined area of injected redness
- Pain
- Watering
- Photophobia

Key observations and findings
- Visual acuity normal

Key actions and treatment
- Self-limiting
- Refer to ophthalmologist
- Oral NSAIDs may help

⑦ Hordeolum stye

Infection of the follicle of an eyelash, usually caused by *Staphylococcus aureus* bacteria.

Key signs and symptoms
- Swelling of the eyelid
- Redness at the edge of the eyelid
- Pain on palpation of the affected area

Key actions and treatment
- Application of warm compresses
- Advise the patient not to touch the stye
- If the stye is touched advise hand washing to prevent spreading the infection
- Avoid eye make-up until resolved

⑦ Subconjunctival haemorrhage

Occurs as the blood vessels in the sclera break due to raised intraocular pressure. It may be spontaneous or occur following coughing, sneezing, lifting heavy objects, straining, or trauma. It looks alarming but is not normally serious.

Key signs and symptoms
- Bright red blood patch on the sclera

Key history and assessment
- Previous trauma

Key observations and findings
- Visual acuity should be normal
- Check BP to ensure no hypertension

Key actions and treatment
- No acute treatment needed, will eventually disperse
- Reassure

Facial problems

Differential diagnosis

True emergencies
- Facial burns
- Maxillary (Le Fort) fractures

Urgent presentations
- Blow out fracture of the orbital floor
- Dislocated mandible
- Epistaxis
- Mandibular fractures
- Nasal injuries
- Tetanus (lockjaw)

① Timely assessment
- Facial wounds

⑦ Non-urgent presentations
- Rhinitis
- Sinusitis

Introduction

The majority of facial problems which present for emergency care are as a result of injury. The main focus of management is to ensure that the airway is not compromised. Facial trauma can be distressing for the patient who may be concerned about the risk of permanent disfigurement. Psychological care of these patients should not be overlooked. Clear explanations of the assessment and treatment should be given. A calm and professional approach will help give confidence to the patient. Avoid giving false reassurance which may later undermine confidence.

☠ Facial burns

Consideration needs to be given to the risk of inhalation injury and the involvement of the airway. The burn itself should be covered with a clean damp cloth as a first aid measure prior to full assessment and treatment.

📖 See Burns and scalds, p.97.

:☠: Maxillary (Le Fort) fractures

Fractures to the middle third of the face were first classified at the turn of the 20th century by Le Fort. Three different fracture patterns (Figs 19.1–3) are recognized as described here. Despite the extent of visible injury it is vital to first ensure the airway is patent and protected.

Le Fort I

A horizontal fracture across the maxilla which runs between the maxillary floor and the orbital floor, above the teeth and palate and below the nose. Results in a floating fragment of the lower maxilla. See Fig. 19.1.

Le Fort II

A pyramidal fracture of the face extending from the apex in the midline at the bridge of the nose, diagonally downwards and outwards involving the medial inferior orbital rims, the zygomatic arches, and the pterygoid bones. See Fig. 19.2.

Le Fort III

A transverse fracture which passes through the orbital ridges, the zygomatic arches, and the superior pterygoid bones. This injury results in a large unstable floating fragment which in effect separates the face from the skull and is sometimes referred to as craniofacial dysjunction. See Fig. 19.3.

'Smash' fractures

Severe comminuted fractures which do not conform to the classic Le Fort patterns are referred to as 'smash' fractures.

Key signs and symptoms

General
- Location of facial wounds
- Facial swelling and bruising which may be extensive
- Pain across the face with areas of local intensity
- Nasopharyngeal bleeding
- Altered facial contours, best visualized by standing behind the patient and looking downwards over the patient's head
- Altered sensation to the check as a result of damage to the infraorbital nerve

Le Fort I
- Bruising of upper lip and lower half of mid-face
- Abnormal mobility of upper teeth and maxilla
- Damage to teeth
- Palpable crepitation above upper lip
- Intra-oral haematomas

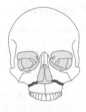 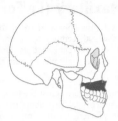

Fig. 19.1 Le Fort fracture lines I

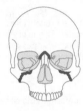 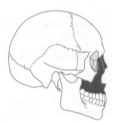

Fig. 19.2 Le Fort fracture lines II

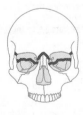 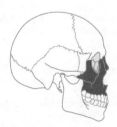

Fig. 19.3 Le Fort fracture lines III

Le Fort II
- Respiratory distress
- Abnormal movement in the maxilla
- Periorbital bruising and haematomas
- Double vision
- Subconjunctival haemorrhage
- CSF rhinorrhoea

Le Fort III
- Respiratory distress
- Middle third of face mobile
- Abnormal movement in the maxilla
- Periorbital bruising and haematomas
- Double vision
- Subconjunctival haemorrhage
- CSF rhinorrhoea

Smash fractures
- Severe comminution of the face
- Associated head injury and other skeletal injuries are highly likely

Key history and assessment
- Assess airway and breathing, ensure airway is patent. Airway problems may develop due to tissue swelling, haemorrhage, vomiting, and loss of gag reflex
- Understand the mechanism of injury to assess the risk of associated injuries
- Assess the potential for head injury

Key observations and findings
- Respiration:
  - observe for tachypnoea and dyspnoea
  - note rate, rhythm, and volume of breathing
- O_2 saturation: ensure levels >94%
- Pulse:
  - tachycardic due to pain or haemorrhage
  - bradycardia may indicate raised intracranial pressure
- Capillary refill: should be <2sec
- BP:
  - regular monitoring required
  - hypertension may be the result of pain; may also indicate rising intracranial pressure
  - hypotensive as a result of hypovolaemia
- Record GCS
- Check pupils for size, equality, and reaction
- Temperature should be recorded as a baseline

Key investigations
- Facial XRs
- CT scan may be required for further facial investigation and/or head/cervical spine injury
- ABG, if any signs of respiratory distress or hypoxia

- FBC, U&E
- Blood glucose
- Group and cross match as required

Key actions and treatments

- Immediate medical and nursing intervention required
- High-flow O_2 via non-rebreathing mask at 15L per min
- Refer to anaesthetist for ongoing airway assessment and management
- Refer to maxillofacial surgeons
- Position patient in a lateral or semi prone position if possible to prevent obstruction of the pharynx by the relaxed lower jaw, tongue, or secretions. *Cervical collar should remain in place until the neck is cleared*
- If other major injuries have been excluded and the patient is able, sit him/her upright leaning forward and encourage secretions and haemorrhage to drain
- Observe for increasing facial swelling
- IV access required (2 large-bore cannulae), IV fluid to maintain BP. Maintain fluid balance chart. May require transfusion
- Observe for confusion: this may be an indicator of hypoxia or raised intracranial pressure
- Assess patient for other problems: scalp lacerations/wounds, low blood sugar etc.
- Apply pressure dressings to bleeding points on head (with a further plan for definitive closure). May require surgical intervention for wound toilet and management
- Consider antibiotic cover according to local guidelines
- Careful provision of IV analgesia to ensure adequate pain relief without depressing respirations or level of consciousness
- Ensure safe transfer to high dependency area, ICU, theatre, or specialist unit

:☼: Blow-out fracture of the orbital floor

This injury usually results from blunt force trauma to the orbit resulting in a sudden increase in pressure within the orbit. A fracture occurs in the thin bone of the orbital floor.

Key signs and symptoms

- Double vision on lateral and upward gaze
- Pain on eye movement
- Periorbital bruising
- Subconjunctival haemorrhage
- Blurred vision
- Reduced or absent sensation over cheek and upper gum

Key history and assessment

- Determine the mechanism of injury to assist in excluding other injuries
- Check pupils for size, equality, and reaction
- Assess visual acuity, visual fields, extrinsic muscle function, external eye structure, anterior eye structures, and fundus
- Assess for indications of head injury
- Check mobility of mandible as posterior displacement or fracture may impair movement
- Check for impairment of sensation below the affected eye and upper gum
- Palpable crepitus (surgical emphysema) may be present around the orbit. *The patient must not blow their nose as this will worsen the situation*
- Displacement of the eyeball and visual loss due to orbital swelling

Key observations and findings

- Observations are usually normal. Tachycardia may result from pain or anxiety. Bradycardia can result from pressure on the eyeball
- Check GCS

Key investigations

- XR may show a fluid level in the maxillary antrum, a 'tear drop' of soft tissue may be seen in the top of the antrum
- CT will provide more detail of a fracture
- Check blood glucose

Key actions and treatments

- Analgesia for pain
- Refer for specialist assessment and management
- If no or minimal fracture displacement is present and no complications are encountered then a conservative approach may be appropriate
- Advise the patient to avoid blowing their nose
- Surgery may be necessary if the displacement is significant

☼ Dislocated mandible

Dislocation of the mandible at the temporomandibular joint (TMJ) may be spontaneous (from a yawn or similar action) or may be due to trauma. Dislocation is normally bilateral but can be unilateral.

Key signs and symptoms
- Inability to close mouth due to the condyles being forced anteriorly
- Considerable pain due to muscle spasm
- Pain on palpation of the masseter muscles

Key history and assessment
- Poor communication due to inability to move jaw and increased pain on attempting to talk
- Take a history from a companion if available
- May need to treat patient prior to obtaining full history
- If the problem is due to trauma, a head injury may need to be excluded, along with any other associated injuries

Key observations and findings
- Pulse, respiratory rate, and BP: may be elevated due to pain and distress

Key investigations
- XR required to exclude fracture following trauma

Key actions and treatments
- Ensure the airway is clear
- IV access required
- Pain relief and sedation may be required to facilitate relocation
- Ensure equipment and personnel available to manage airway if necessary
- To reduce the jaw, the healthcare practitioner faces the patient and places an object such an oropharyngeal airway, or a padded tongue depressor partially in the patient's mouth to prevent their jaw snapping closed. The thumbs are placed on the lower posterior teeth, while the fingers move the inferior border of the mandible downwards and then backwards. A click should be felt with the joint relocates
- If sedated, observe patient until fully conscious and alert
- Advice should be given regarding: follow-up care, soft diet for at least a week, stifle yawns, support jaw if yawning, avoid wide opening
- Refer to maxillofacial surgeon for follow-up

☼ Epistaxis

Bleeding from the nose is common, occurring most frequently in children and the elderly. The majority of bleeds occur from the anterior septum and are easier to control than posterior haemorrhage which tends to be more severe. A significant epistaxis can be extremely distressing. So called 'digital trauma' (nose picking) is the most common cause. Direct blows to the nose, irritation of the mucosa due to infection or inflammation may also trigger bleeding. Epistaxis is more common in hypertensive patients.

Key signs and symptoms
- Obvious nasal haemorrhage

Key history and assessment
- Action to stop active bleeding should occur before the taking of a detailed history
- How long has it been bleeding?
- Have any clots been passed?
- Which side is bleeding?
- History of trauma
- Previous episodes
- Current medications: especially anticoagulants, NSAIDs
- Relevant past medical history: e.g. hypertension, bleeding disorder, previous nasal problems
- Pain
- Is the bleed uncontrollable or controllable with pressure?
- If traumatic, any associated injuries, especially head or neck?
- Allergies
- Recent URTI

Key observations and findings
- Pulse: may be tachycardic due to anxiety or blood loss
- BP: may be hypertensive due to pre-existing condition or anxiety. Hypotension should trigger urgent review and consideration of the need for fluid resuscitation
- Respiratory rate: may be tachypnoeic due to anxiety
- SpO_2: should be normal
- Temperature: may be increased if recent infection

Key investigations
- None normally required if bleeding stops easily with direct pressure
- If significant haemorrhage or other concurrent medical problem
- FBC, U&E, INR if on warfarin

Key actions and treatments
- Assess airway and breathing
- Ensure the patient is haemodynamically stable, if not commence fluid resuscitation, high-flow O_2 and obtain senior medical assistance
- If the patient is stable and still bleeding:
  - make the patient as comfortable as possible
  - have them blow their nose to remove any clots

- lean the patient forward and encourage them to spit any blood out of their mouth rather than swallowing it
- apply direct pressure to both sides of the nose just below the nasal bone. If possible apply a swimmer's clip which provides constant, even pressure. This should be left in situ for at least 20min to ensure clotting occurs but for not >30min to prevent pressure damage occurring
- reassess for bleeding on removal of clip
- reassess pulse, respiratory rate and BP prior to discharge to ensure tachycardia or tachypnoea has resolved. Patients with long-standing hypertension may be discharged following medical review
- patients who are hypotensive should have senior medical review
- The nostril may need to be packed using a nasal tampon. Refer for pack removal according to local guidelines—normally after 48 hours
- If bleeding continues despite treatment, refer to ENT surgeons for further assessment and consideration of cauterization
- Offer frequent mouthwashes to clean and remove any blood particles
- Observe for signs of increased restlessness which may indicate hypovolaemia
- If discharging home advise the patient to refrain from any hot drinks, alcohol, or blowing the nose
- Advise to seek assistance immediately should the bleeding recommence

:☼: Mandibular fractures

Fractures of the mandible normally occur as a result of direct force to the jaw during an assault, sport, or road traffic collision.

Key signs and symptoms
- Pain in the lower jaw or teeth
- Difficulty in speaking
- Difficulty in swallowing
- Dribbling of blood-stained fluid due to haemorrhages/cuts within the mouth
- Facial deformity
- Teeth misaligned
- Bruising under the tongue

Key history and assessment
- Ensure airway is patent and protected
- Determine the mechanism of injury to enable associated injuries to be excluded, particularly head and cervical spine injuries
- Assess ability to fully open mouth and to clench teeth. If this is normal then the risk of mandible fracture is low
- If one mandible fracture is seen a second fracture or dislocation is normally present

Key observations and findings
- Pulse: may be tachycardic due to pain or anxiety
- Respiratory rate: should be normal
- BP: should be normal but may be hypertensive due to pain or anxiety
- Check GCS

Key investigations
- XR to identify structural bony problems. Orthopantomograms (OPGs) if available are the most useful

Key actions and treatments
- Ensure airway is maintained
- IV access required for analgesia
- IV fluids may be needed due to maintain hydration if poor oral intake
- Antibiotics if fracture is compound in accordance with local guidelines
- Refer to maxillofacial surgeon

☼ Nasal injuries

Nasal fractures are very common. Presentation may be at the time of the incidence due to bleeding or pain, or later due to deformity or difficulty breathing.

Key signs and symptoms
- Obvious trauma to the nose
- Epistaxis

Key history and assessment
- Obtain a clear history of the mechanism of injury to evaluate the risk of associated injuries
- Assess the extent of any nasal deformity. Give the patient a mirror to allow them to assess the injury as a deformity may not be new
- Check for septal deviation and septal haematoma by inspecting the nasal airways. Septal haematomas may lead to avascular necrosis of the cartilage and possible collapse of the bridge
- Associated zygomatic and orbital fractures may be present. A full eye examination should be undertaken
- Assess for leakage of CSF which indicates a base of skull fracture

Key observations and findings
- Pulse, respiratory rate, and BP should all be normal, however they may be tachycardic, tachypnoeic, or hypertensive due to distress
- SpO_2 should be normal

Key investigations
- None required
- XR is not helpful unless associated facial fractures are suspected

Key actions and treatments
- Ensure airway is patent
- Manage any active bleeding as described—🕮 see Epistaxis, p.211
- Arrange for ENT review if required according to local practice after 48–72 hours to allow for initial swelling to subside
- Provide oral analgesia
- Advise against drinking alcohol, hot drinks, or blowing nose

:⚙: Tetanus (lockjaw)

Although rare in developed countries with mass vaccination programmes, where 5 vaccinations provide a lifetime's cover, tetanus is still responsible for a number of deaths each year, with mortality rate of around 60% if untreated. The condition is caused by a neurotoxin produced by the anaerobic bacteria *Clostridium tetani*. The bacteria forms spores which may lie dormant for long periods in soil and animal faeces. They contaminate the body by entering via a wound or burn, with deep or grossly contaminated wounds presenting the highest risk, although even small puncture wounds may be enough to allow the spores to enter. The incubation period is normally between 3 days and 3 weeks although it can develop very quickly given the right circumstances or take several months before clinical signs are visible.

Key signs and symptoms
- Headache
- Sore throat
- Spasm of the muscles adjacent to the wound
- Progression to painful spasms and rigid clamping of the jaw—lockjaw
- Difficulty swallowing due to spasm of the throat
- Difficulty breathing due to chest wall spasm
- Eventually all skeletal muscles may become involved
- Spasms may become painful and exhausting
- Sensitivity to touch
- Seizures

Key history and assessment
- History of wound in previous days or weeks
- If unable to recall wound, any history of exposure to area or activity of risk such farm visit, close contact with animals, gardening, outdoors sports
- Assess extent of muscle spasm
- Assess airway and gag reflex
- Assess effectiveness of respirations
- Assess for development of septicaemia

Key observations and findings
- Temperature: pyrexial
- Pulse: tachycardia
- Respiratory rate: tachypnoea and dyspnoea
- BP: often hypotensive
- Observe for loss of gag reflex
- Observe for excessive secretions in mouth due to difficulty in swallowing
- O_2 saturation
- Check capillary refill: should be <2sec
- Observe peripheries and lips for signs of cyanosis

Key investigations
- Normally diagnosed from history and signs and symptoms
- Blood microbiology to confirm infection
- FBC, U&Es, blood glucose, ABGs

Key actions and treatments
- *Obtain senior medical assistance immediately*
- Airway and breathing:
  - manage jaw position, tongue, and secretions to prevent airway occlusion. Place patient in a lateral or semi prone position
  - O_2 via a non-rebreathing mask at 15L per min
  - consideration will need to be given to anaesthetizing the patient to protect the airway and maintain adequate oxygenation
  - tracheostomy may be required due to laryngeal spasm and allows respiratory assistance and a way of suctioning secretions
- IV access required: 2 large-bore cannulae
- IV benzodiazepine such as diazepam to relax muscle spasm
- Observe for restlessness: may be an indicator of hypoxia
- Antibiotic therapy, according to local guidelines
- Tetanus immunoglobulin
- IV fluids and maintain fluid balance chart
- Protect patient from injury due to muscle spasm and cognitive impaired function with the use of bed sides and additional pillows or padding
- Manage pyrexia which occurs due to increased metabolic rate from muscle spasm. Maintain pressure area care for skin integrity. Monitor Waterlow score
- Transfer to high dependency area—ICU/HDU
- Tetanus is a notifiable disease in the UK

ⓘ Facial wounds

Wounds to the face require special consideration due to the relationship of the skin to the facial muscles which can make it difficult to close lacerations without leaving a deformity. The need for an acceptable cosmetic result in all patients should mean referral to plastic surgery occurs in all but the simplest of lacerations.

📖 See Wounds, p.427.

ⓘ Rhinitis

Inflammation of the nasal mucous membrane is one of the most common conditions experienced. It occurs as a symptom of the common cold and in allergic reactions. Excessive mucus production occurs causing the familiar 'runny nose'. Soft tissues become swollen, blocking air passage through the nasal cavity leading to a feeling of a blocked nose. Emergency care may be sought if the condition has been persisting longer than the patient expects.

Key signs and symptoms
- Rhinorrhoea—runny nose
- Inability to breathe freely through the nasal passages
- Sneezing
- Irritation of the nose
- Accompanying sore throat
- Watering, itchy eye

Key history and assessment
- History should be focused towards excluding any serious complications or underlying conditions
- For allergic rhinitis: exposure to potential allergens

Key observations and findings
- Check temperature, pulse, respiratory rate, all may be slightly raised in viral rhinitis depending upon the extent of the infection. In allergic rhinitis expect all to be within normal parameters

Key investigations
- None normally required

Key actions and treatments
- No specific treatment for viral rhinitis
- Advise that the condition should resolve within 5–7 days
- OTC preparations are available to assist in coping with the symptoms
- Oral antihistamines may help with allergic rhinitis as may steroidal nasal sprays
- Avoiding the allergen is the most effective management although this may not be possible if pollen or another widely distributed substance is the trigger

⑦ Sinusitis

Infection of the sinuses is relatively common. Emergency care is normally sought for pain control. The maxillary sinuses which lie behind each cheek are most frequently affected, but it can affect the ethmoid and frontal sinuses. The condition is normally precipitated by a viral upper respiratory infection. The resulting inflammation of the sinuses causes excessive mucus production and blockage of the drainage followed by a secondary bacterial infection. As secretions accumulate in the sinuses the increase in pressure causes pain.

Key signs and symptoms
- Facial pain: increases on palpation over the affected sinuses
- Pain may be positional: worse when lying down
- Headache
- Pain in the jaw: worse on movement
- Toothache in the upper teeth
- General malaise
- Rhinitis

Key history and assessment
- History of a recent URTI
- Pre-existing risk factors:
  - allergies
  - nasal polyp
  - smoking
  - asthma
  - immunocompromised
  - cystic fibrosis
  - pregnancy

Key observations and findings
- Check temperature, pulse, and respiratory rate

Key investigations
- None required

Key actions and treatment
- The majority of cases resolve without healthcare intervention within 5–7 days
- Simple analgesic such as paracetamol, aspirin, or NSAIDs will help manage the pain and pyrexia
- Antibiotics may be required if the symptoms persist beyond a week
- Nasal decongestants may provide temporary relief from a blocked nose but continued use beyond 3–5 days may worsen the condition
- Advise the patient to rest. Lying supine can increase the pain, sitting upright in a chair or lying in a lateral position may be more acceptable
- Advise the patient to increase fluid intake—warm drinks are best as cold fluid may cause the pain to increase
- Steam inhalations have no proven benefit. However some patients do report temporary relief of symptoms. A hot shower is the most

practical way of generating steam while minimizing the risk of scalding. Similarly the application of a warm cloth over the sinuses may provide some relief
- Follow-up in primary care if no improvement after a week or if recurrent condition

Falls

Differential diagnosis

True emergencies
- Falls from a height

Timely assessment
- Slips, trips, and falls

Introduction

The presentation of a patient following a fall is one of the most common reasons for requiring emergency care. In people >65 years old falls are the commonest cause of death from injury. Falls may result from many causes (Box 20.1):

Box 20.1 Possible causes of falls

Medical	Environmental
• Alcohol or drug intoxication	• Bad lighting
• Alzheimer's disease	• Uneven or damaged pavements
• Cardiac arrhythmias	• Obstructions
• Cardiac arrest	• Worn or slippery flooring
• Hypoglycaemia	• Ill-fitting footwear
• Labyrinthitis	• Inappropriate walking aids
• Multiple medications (>4)	• Poor work practice at height
• Parkinson's disease	• Overstretching
• Psychotropic medications	• Poor work equipment
• Stroke	• Leisure activities, climbing, etc.
• Visual problems	

Injuries resulting from a fall range from minor soft tissue injuries to those which are serious or life threatening. The presence of one obvious injury should not distract the examiner from ensuring a thorough examination is performed in order to avoid missing other injuries. In the elderly, fractured necks of femur may be missed in patients who are still able to mobilize.

☠ Falls from a height

Falls from a height are a major cause of serious injury. In the UK one person per week dies as a result of falling from a height, with >60 people being seriously injured. The extent of the injury depends on the distance fallen, the surface the patient impacts on, whether or not they hit any obstruction during the fall, and the position they land in. Serious injury or death may occur following falls from a relatively low height with 60% of victims falling from a height of 2m or lower.

Assessment should follow major trauma management guidelines: commence with a primary survey, resuscitation, a secondary survey, and then definitive treatment.

① Slips, trips, and falls

Commonly a presentation seen in older people, slips, trips, and falls are also the most common workplace accidents. The first priority in assessment should be to determine the exact mechanism of the accident in order to ascertain whether the fall resulted from a simple slip, trip, or an underlying medical condition. A thorough history from the patient and, if possible, from any witnesses is required.

Once injuries resulting from the fall have been treated, consideration should be given to the reason the patient fell and what action can be taken to prevent a reoccurrence. Assessment of elderly patients who have experienced a fall should include observation of balance and gait.

If the fall is a recurrent event or if there are any doubts regarding the cause, patients should be offered a referral to a specialist falls service.

Further reading

National Institute for Clinical Excellence (2004). Clinical Guideline 21. The assessment and prevention of falls on older people. NICE. London

Fits

Differential diagnosis

True emergencies

- Hypoglycaemia
- Status epilepticus

Urgent presentations

- Epilepsy

Timely assessment

- Pseudoseizures

Introduction

Alternatively referred to as convulsions or seizures, fits are a symptom not a condition. Patients often present as an emergency due to the sudden spontaneous onset and anxiety the fit may cause in witnesses. Fits occur as a result of sudden disorganized electrical activity in the brain. They normally last between 30sec and 2min. The effect upon the individual will depend on the area and extent of the brain involved. Most authors prefer the term 'seizure' as the word 'fit' has differing connotations; 'to have a fit' may be used to describe anger or loss of temper. There are many causes of seizures which can be classified into five main groups:

1. Cerebral irritation
- Infection: meningitis, encephalitis
- Head injury
- Poisoning:
  - drug reaction/overdose, both prescription medications and illicit drugs
  - venomous bites and stings
- Space-occupying lesions—tumour, abscess
- Photosensitive triggers—video games, flashing lights
- Electric shock
- Heat stroke
- Uraemia

2. Metabolic disorders
- Hypoxia—airway obstruction, cardiac dysrhythmias, respiratory arrest
- Hypoglycaemia
- Hyponatraemia

3. Substance withdrawal
- Alcohol
- Barbiturates
- Opiates

4. Idiopathic

5. Pseudo-seizures
Regardless of the classification all seizures require a consistent approach to assessment.

Key signs and symptoms
The symptoms of seizures vary widely between individual patients. They may include:
- Collapse
- Muscle spasms with twitching and jerking limbs
- Excessive salivation
- Incontinence
- Disorientation
- Abnormal eye movements
- Grunting
- Teeth clenching and grinding

- Unusual mannerisms—rubbing skin, twitching finger, picking at clothing
- Labile emotional states—sudden anger, laughter, crying
- Hallucinations

Key actions and treatment

- Prevent further injury from falling or banging against objects, but do not try to restrain them or place anything into their mouth
- Place the patient into the recovery position as soon as the seizure stops
- Be aware the patient may be very confused and frightened when coming around—post-ictal state

☠ Hypoglycaemia

Patients with diabetes who develop severe hypoglycaemia may present in an unconscious state which can lead to epileptiform seizures. These appear like epilepsy but are due to a secondary condition and not bio-electrical activity. If the blood glucose is low and the patient unconscious IM glucagon or IV glucose should be given accordingly.

📖 See Diabetes, p.157.

☠ Status epilepticus

Status epilepticus is defined as a continuous, generalized, convulsive seizure lasting >20min or a series of seizures between which the patient does not regain consciousness. The condition is considered a medical emergency as it is associated with significant morbidity and mortality.

Key signs and symptoms
- Seizure lasting >20min
- Failure to regain consciousness between seizures

Key history and assessment
- Treatment should be commenced immediately
- Obtain a history from witnesses if possible
- Ascertain whether any treatment has been given e.g. rectal diazepam
- Consider causes such as poor compliance with medication, alcohol withdrawal, or metabolic disorders

Key observations
- *Do not delay treatment to record observations*
- If possible, observe respiratory rate, pulse, SpO_2, temperature, and BP: these may need to be performed manually
- Repeat observations at least every 15min

Key investigations
- Blood glucose
- U&Es, anti-convulsant levels if available

Key actions and treatment
- Protect the patient from further harm
- Drug therapy: rectal diazepam or buccal midazolam may be given in community settings and sometimes by non-healthcare professionals who have been trained in its application. Effective in 70% of cases
- If ineffective:
  - IV glucose 50mL of 50% if blood glucose low
  - IV lorazepam 1.5-2.5mg—this can be repeated *once* after 10min
- If ineffective: phenytoin infusion 15–18mg/kg at 50mg/min
- If patient is still fitting: urgent anaesthetics assessment
- Identify and treat any underlying medical problems
- Admit to critical care environment

☼ Epilepsy

Epilepsy is thought to affect approximately 2% of the population. It is defined as the presence of recurrent intermittent seizures which are not related to a current medical condition. It should be remembered that epilepsy is a medical condition rather than a label. A single seizure does not mean the patient has epilepsy. The diagnosis should only be made by a neurologist following investigation. All patients should have an agreed care plan.

In around 75% of cases, there is no known cause: in the remaining 25%, the most common causes are:
- Head injury
- Complication of cerebral infection
- Fetal brain injury
- Hypoxic birth injury
- Side effect of substance misuse or environmental poisoning
- Brain tumour
- Stroke

Classification of seizures

Previous classifications of seizures such as grand or petit mal are no longer recommended. Attempts have been made to agree international classifications and currently >40 different types of epilepsy are recognized. The more common presentations include:

Partial seizures
- Simple partial (focal) seizures:
  - patient remains aware
  - rigidity in limbs or face
  - limbs twitch on one side only
  - patient experiences altered sensations, strange smells, visual changes
  - altered emotions
- Complex partial (focal) seizures:
  - aura before the seizure starts
  - loss of awareness
  - automatisms, chewing motion, repetitive actions
  - unresponsive to verbal commands
  - loss of consciousness

Generalized seizures
- Tonic-clonic seizure:
  - collapse
  - loss of consciousness
  - rigidity of body
  - uncontrollable limb movement
  - tongue biting
  - incontinence
- Absence seizures:
  - last <10sec
  - staring
  - lack of awareness

- twitching of muscles
- rapid eyelid movement
- Myoclonic seizures:
  - sudden violent jerking of a limb or torso
  - no loss of consciousness
- Atonic seizures:
  - sudden relaxation of muscles
  - collapse or uncontrollable head drop
  - loss of consciousness

Key history and assessment

- Is the patient known to have epilepsy?
- When was their last seizure?
- Any known trigger factors?
- How long did this seizure last?
- Any auras before the seizure?
- Any symptoms afterwards—headache, vomiting, disorientation?
- Any associated factors—diabetes, change in medication, alcohol?
- Any systemic infections?
- Any injuries?
- Witnessed or unwitnessed?
- Was this seizure similar to previous ones? If not, in what way was it different?

Key observations and findings

- Baseline temperature, pulse, respiratory rate, and BP: all should be normal

Key investigations

- None required for single episodes which fit an existing pattern
- If increasing frequency or unusual presentation, FBC, U&Es, glucose, ECG

Key actions and treatments

- If the seizure resolves spontaneously within 5min, follows the patient's usual pattern, and they are fully alert and orientated, there is no indication for any intervention
- Other presentations:
  - may require specialist referral
  - follow-up should be arranged in line with local procedures
- Post-ictal care:
  - some patients will become fully alert and orientated almost immediately, others may take 30min or longer—particularly if given benzodiazepines
  - during this time they may have a reduced GCS and be disorientated, confused, wandering, frightened, or aggressive
  - patients should be accompanied during this period to prevent harm and to help them become reorientated
- Patients should not be discharged until fully alert, orientated, and accompanied

First seizure

Anyone experiencing a first seizure should be referred to a specialist in the management of epilepsy if no reversible causes are found at initial presentation. The presence of any focal signs warrant consideration of a CT scan. Anticonvulsant therapy should not be started until the diagnosis of epilepsy is confirmed. If the patient is to be discharged a full neurological examination must be completed. The patient, and any appropriate companion, should be given information on how to recognize a seizure, what action to take, and the importance of reporting any more seizures. The patient should be advised not to drive or operate machinery and to report the event to the Driver and Vehicle Licensing Agency (DVLA).

ⓘ **Pseudoseizures**

Referred to as non-epileptic attack disorder, this presentation is common and can be difficult to distinguish from epileptic seizures. However, pseudoseizures are relatively common in patients who also suffer from epilepsy. Indicators of pseudoseizures include:

- Patient resists examination
- Patient calls out during the seizure
- Patient remains conscious whilst having bilateral limb contractions

Further reading

National Institute for Clinical Excellence (2004). *Clinical Guideline 20: Epilepsy. The epilepsies: the diagnosis and management of the epilepsies in adults and children in primary and secondary care.* London: NICE.

Foreign bodies

Differential diagnosis

☺ True emergency
- Airway obstruction

☼ Urgent presentations
- Foreign bodies in throat
- Impalement

① Timely assessment
- Genital and rectal foreign bodies
- Foreign bodies in the eye
- Ingestion of foreign body
- Nasal foreign bodies

⑦ Non urgent presentations
- Aural foreign bodies
- Superficial soft tissue foreign bodies

Introduction

Presentations of FBs are extremely varied, ranging from major life-threatening events such as airway obstruction to everyday occurrences like splinters. It is important to ensure each patient is treated according to their individual circumstances. Mismanagement of even the most simple presentations may lead to complications which can result in weeks of pain and discomfort.

☠ Airway obstruction

Airway obstruction is a life-threatening emergency. Immediate medical assistance is required.

Key signs and symptoms
- Coughing
- Difficulty breathing
- Stridor
- Cyanosis
- Confusion
- Drowsiness
- Respiratory arrest

Key history and assessment
- Do not delay treatment in order to obtain history when patient has respiratory distress
- History from patient or witness if possible

Key observations and findings
- Do not delay treatment in order to record clinical observations when patient is in respiratory distress
- Breathing may be noisy—stridor
- Respiratory rate may be fast, slow or absent depending on severity of presentation
- SpO_2 may be low: <94% on air
- Pulse: patient may have tachycardia, bradycardia, or cardiac arrest
- Record GCS/AVPU: may be reduced

Key investigations
- None

Key actions and treatment
- Call for immediate medical assistance
- Perform basic airway manoeuvres
- O_2 via a non-rebreathing mask
- Remove clearly visible obstructions if possible
- *DO NOT persevere if object is difficult to remove*: risk of complete obstruction
- Attempt to ventilate with bag/valve/mask device if respiratory arrest occurs

:✪: Foreign bodies in throat

This is a common presentation and in adults is usually due to fish or chicken bones, or a meat bolus. The FB is likely to be found in the crico-pharynx, the oesophagus, or the gastro-oesophageal junction. Fish bones can lodge in the tonsil or at the back of the tongue.

Key signs and symptoms
- Difficulty breathing suggests airway obstruction
- Dysphagia
- Drooling
- Retching
- FB sensation

Key history and assessment
- Determine if airway is threatened
- Note timing of onset of symptoms, especially in relation to eating
- Assess ability to swallow
- Recent throat infection: swelling may cause dysphagia

Key observations and findings
- Respiratory rate:
  - tachypnoea
  - dyspnoea
- O_2 saturation: should be normal unless airway or breathing is compromised
- Pulse: may be tachycardic due to distress
- BP: may be hypertensive due to distress
- Cardiac monitoring: indicated if airway compromised
- Visible FB may be present

Key investigations
- If the FB is radio-opaque, lateral XR of the neck may be helpful in iden-tifying FBs such as coins and large fish bones

Key actions and treatment
- Place patient in a position comfortable for them without compromising their airway
- If the patient is not distressed, can swallow saliva, is not drooling, and FB is visible:
  - Spencer Wells forceps can be used to remove FB
  - may need more than one attempt
  - vomit bowl and suction should be at hand in case of retching and vomiting
  - if FB successfully removed check the patient can swallow without difficulty prior to discharge
  - advice should be given regarding oral hygiene
  - simple analgesia
- If the FB is not successfully removed then refer to ENT

:✪: Impalement

Becoming impaled on an object can occur following a road traffic collision, a fall from a height, during sport, or as part of an assault.

📖 See Major trauma, p.293.

Key signs and symptoms
- Do not be distracted by the patient's presentation from undertaking a full primary survey

Key history and assessment
- Understanding of the mechanism of injury is required:
  - how long ago did the incident occur?
  - duration of impalement
  - any history of entrapment?
- Events prior to incident:
  - dizziness
  - loss of consciousness
  - intoxication
  - seizure
- Entry site
- Assess distal circulation, sensation, and function
- Assess extent of blood loss
- Any other injuries?
- Relevant past medical history
- Consider potential for criminal or health and safety investigation and the need to retain evidence

Key observations and findings
- Breathing:
  - rate
  - adequacy
- Pulse may be raised due to pain or blood loss
- BP should be recorded
- Regular neurological observations: every 15min for early changes in conscious level and motor or sensory changes
- Continuous cardiac monitoring for arrhythmias

Key investigations
- XR may be helpful to determine location and nature of object
- Urgent CT scan may be required to exclude injury to underlying structures
- ABGs: if any signs of respiratory distress or hypoxia
- FBC and U&Es: baseline measurements
- Group or cross match according to clinical condition

Key actions and treatments
- *Do not attempt to remove the object* before assessment by senior clinician and appropriate facilities are available. This is likely to require a fully staffed operating theatre
- Secure object if the patient has to be transferred

- Position patient in a position comfortable for them without compromising the impaled area or increasing pain
- IV access: 2 large-bore cannulas
- If any signs of airway obstruction or shock are present:
  - immediate experienced medical assistance
  - high-flow O_2 via non-rebreathing mask
  - fluid as required to maintain adequate BP
- Maintain fluid balance chart
- Apply pressure dressing to any bleeding points
- Consider prophylactic antibiotics for contaminated wounds
- Check tetanus status and administer according to protocol
- Pain relief as guided by the patient's condition

① Genital and rectal foreign bodies

A range of objects may present as an emergency having been inserted and lost in the urethra, vagina, or rectum. It is important to recognize the embarrassment which may be caused to the patient. Wherever possible the healthcare professional should be the same gender as the patient and privacy should be maintained at all times. It is advisable for the examiner to be chaperoned. The healthcare professional should not be judgemental in any way. Occasionally, insertion may be an act of self-harm and this should be addressed. The possibility of abuse should also be considered.

Key signs and symptoms
- Visible FB
- Pain
- Loss of function
- Bleeding

Key history and assessment
- Sometimes the history will be vague due to embarrassment
- Try to speak to the patient without relatives present if appropriate
- Consider potential sexual assault and abuse
- Pain: note location, extent, and type. Abdominal pain may indicate perforation

Key observations and findings
- If FB in situ for several days, TPR for signs of infection or toxic shock syndrome

Key investigations
- XR investigation may be required depending on the object and location
- Endoscopy may also be required

Key actions and treatment
- Rectal FBs: often require removal under a general anaesthetic (GA) due to sphincter spasm and the requirement to ensure no damage has been caused to the bowel
- Urethral FB: often require removal under GA
- Vaginal FB: gynecological referral for investigation and removal

① Foreign bodies in the eye

Ocular FBs are very common. The vast majority will be removed without the involvement of a healthcare professional. Those which do present for professional help will be either serious penetrating eye injuries or smaller FBs which are causing the patient discomfort or visual problems. In most cases attempts will have been made to remove the object already and consideration must be given to any damage these may have caused.

📖 See Eye problems, p.169.

ⓘ Ingestion of foreign body

Many strange things are ingested—this may be accidental or as an act of self-harm. If the FB passes through to the stomach it is likely to pass through the GI tract without any complications. Button batteries can cause significant problems if passage through the GI tract is delayed—leakage of caustic contents and electrical current leakage may result in injury. Open safety pins can cause particular problems and often require endoscopic removal. Small button magnets which can be found on children's toys may cause significant damage to the GI tract as a result of pressure necrosis and perforation and therefore require medical assessment.

Key signs and symptoms
- Often no signs or symptoms
- Minor signs and symptoms:
  - pain in throat
  - painful swallowing
  - FB sensation in throat
  - blood in the mouth
- Major signs and symptoms:
  - drooling
  - haematemesis
  - vomiting
  - dysphagia
  - abdominal pain

Key history and assessment
- Identification of FB
- Timing of ingestion
- Events relating to ingestion
- Psychiatric history if relevant

Key observations and findings
- None normally required
- Evidence of previous self-harm

Key investigations
- Radio-opaque FB:
  - XR neck and chest to check the FB is not lodged in the oesophagus
  - metal objects may be located with a metal detector

Key actions and treatment
- The majority of objects will pass without any intervention
- Do not make the patient vomit
- Do not give laxatives
- Simple analgesia for a sore throat if the object has been swallowed
- If abdominal pain or haematemesis are present refer to surgeons
- Referral to mental health services for assessment if appropriate

① Nasal foreign bodies

These are rare in adults. If present try having the patient close the unaffected nostril by placing a finger against the outside and pressing it against the midline and then exhale forcefully down the affected nostril to dislodge the FB. If visible the FB may be removed by sitting the patient upright and carefully passing a blunt hook or loop beyond the object and gently pulling it down. Any difficulties in removal should lead to an ENT referral. Once removed the nostrils should be examined to exclude the presence of septal haematomas. Consideration should be given to the risk of inhalation at all times.

⑦ Aural foreign bodies

The most common aural FB in adult is a cotton bud used by the patient in an attempt to remove wax from the ear canal. Erasers from the ends of pencils are also seen. Insects may also fly into the ear and become stuck. Ear piercings may also become embedded—normally in the lobe but on occasion piercings in the cartilage may work themselves under the skin.

Key signs and symptoms
- History of FB in ear
- Discharge from ear
- Reduction in hearing
- Palpable FB in earlobe or under skin

Key history and assessment
- History may be vague if the patient is embarrassed by their actions
- If embedded FB:
  - what is the object?
  - how long has the object been embedded?

Key actions and treatments
- Attempt to visualize.
  - FB may be removed with alligator forceps or loops
  - extreme care required to ensure no damage is caused to the tympanic membrane
- Insects:
  - instillation of olive oil will kill the insect to allow removal
  - ensure all of the insect is removed
- Following removal from ear canal ensure tympanic membrane is intact
- Advice to patient regarding aural hygiene—cotton buds should not be used to remove wax
- If FB is not easily removed then refer to ENT: does not need to be immediate, referral can wait overnight
- Piercings:
  - remove from behind using splinter forceps, may need nitrous oxide/ oxygen (Entonox®) or LA to facilitate removal
  - ensure thorough cleaning of wound
  - advice on wound healing

⑦ Superficial soft tissue foreign bodies

Splinters of materials such as wood, glass, metal, or plastic are extremely common. FBs such as air gun pellets may occur as the result of illegal activity and consideration will need to be given to reporting such incidents and the management of potential evidence.

Key signs and symptoms
- FB sensation
- Discomfort/pain
- Visible FB
- Signs of inflammation or infection
- Entry wound

Key history and assessment
- History of FB:
  - mechanism of injury
  - timing of injury
  - material involved
  - location and relevant anatomy
- Assessment:
  - joint pain
  - potential for tendon damage
- Allergies
- Tetanus status
- Signs of infection

Key observations and findings
- Distal pulse and sensation should be recorded before and after removal
- Range of movement in relevant joints should be noted

Key investigations
- XR may be required if the FB is not visible and it is thought to be radio-opaque
- A marker, such as a open paper clip taped to the skin, should be used as a point of reference

Key actions and treatments
- The removal of even the most obvious of FB must not be attempted lightly. An assessment of the potential risks and complications must be undertaken prior to any action being taken
- If visible or obviously palpable:
  - adequate analgesia and local/regional anaesthesia should be provided
  - stable, well-lit procedure field required
  - an incision perpendicular to the entry wound may be the most effective method of removal
  - following removal, reassessment must be undertaken to ensure complete removal
  - movement and sensation should be rechecked and documented following removal
  - all wounds should be cleaned and dressed appropriately
  - written and verbal advice should be given

- If not visible or palpable: obtain a senior medical opinion. Do not go 'fishing'
- If the FB may have penetrated a joint space referral for orthopaedic opinion is required
- FBs in hands or feet can be extremely difficult to remove and carry a high risk of additional damage being caused during exploration for removal
- Splinters under fingernails may be removed easily if the end of the object can be cleanly held. More often than not however, attempts by the patient to remove the object themselves have resulted in this proving very difficult to do. The splinter may be accessed by scraping away the overlying nail with a scalpel blade or if deeply embedded, the nail itself may have to be removed. Nitrous oxide/oxygen (Entonox®) and/or a ring block may be required to facilitate these procedures
- Barbed FBs require adequate LA before the object is pushed through and the barbs cut off before removal

Gastrointestinal bleed

Differential diagnosis

True emergencies
- Major bleed with cardiovascular compromise
- Oesophageal varices

Urgent presentations
- Gastrointestinal bleed without cardiovascular compromise

Introduction

Bleeding from the GI tract can be either from the small or large bowel.

Potential causes of upper GI bleeding

- Acute gastritis
- Ingestion of corrosive substances
- Mallory–Weiss tear
- Oesophageal varices
- Peptic ulceration
- Ruptured oesophagus

Potential causes of lower GI bleeding

- Anal fissure
- Colitis
- Colorectal cancer
- Constipation
- Diverticular disease
- Haemorrhoids

Upper GI bleeding may present with either of two main symptoms—haematemesis or melaena. The vomiting of blood (haematemesis) should give rise to concern and prompt immediate medical review. The type and quantity of bleeding should be noted. This can range from a small number of red flecks to a major life-threatening bleed. Emergency treatment is required as delay may result in hypovolaemia and cardiovascular collapse. Vomiting of dark, granular 'coffee-ground' material can indicate the presence of blood which has been in the stomach for some time and which has been partially digested. The passage of melaena (black, tarry, offensive-smelling stools) indicates an upper GI bleed, where the blood has been digested during transit through the bowel.

Lower GI bleeding can occur from the colon, rectum, or anus. The majority of episodes are minor and self-limiting. Patients may notice a few drops of blood when wiping themselves; others may report passing clots along with stool. In severe cases large quantities of fresh blood may be passed. Treatment depends on the severity of bleeding and can range from advice about diet and avoiding constipation to fluid resuscitation and emergency transfusion.

Major trauma may also cause GI bleeding and should be excluded in these patients. Sexual assault should be considered in traumatic bleeding with no other obvious cause.

Chronic GI bleeding may result in iron deficiency anaemia resulting in the patient feeling tired, lethargic, and weak. The bleeding may not be visible to the naked eye and faecal occult blood testing may be required.

☠ Major bleed with cardiovascular compromise

These patients usually present with obvious signs of GI bleeding—this includes haematemesis, obvious rectal blood loss, and collapse. Treatment follows the principles of cardiovascular resuscitation.

Key signs and symptoms

- Haematemesis: fresh blood or coffee-ground vomit
- Fresh blood PR
- Melaena
- Restlessness and anxiety
- Altered conscious level
- Pale, cold, and clammy
- Collapse

Key history and assessment

- Peptic ulcer disease
- Known liver disease
- Trauma

Key observations and findings

- Pulse: rapid, thready, weak, irregular due to hypovolaemia
- Cardiac monitoring is required
- BP: hypotension, may be unrecordable due to blood volume loss and shifting of blood volume to vital organs therefore observe for pale, clammy skin
- Respiratory rate: tachypnoea, dyspnoea
- O_2 saturation: may be difficult to record if hypovolaemia present
- Monitor and record GCS

Key investigations

- ABGs
- FBC, U&Es, glucose, LFTs, clotting factors
- Urgent cross match

Key actions and treatment

- Immediate medical support
- Maintain airway and breathing:
  - ensure patent airway
  - remove blood/vomitus with a wide-bore suction catheter
  - O_2 administered via non-rebreathing mask at 15L
- Emergency anaesthetic assessment if reduced GCS or patient requiring urgent transfer to theatre
- IV access with wide-bore cannula ×2
- IV fluids and blood transfusion according to local guidelines/medical advice
- Medical/surgical referral as appropriate
- Vasoconstrictor drug therapy (e.g. terlipressin) may be required for variceal bleeds
- Catheterization and hourly monitoring for fluid balance control
- Provide clear explanation to patients

:☠: **Oesophageal varices**

Chronic hepatic disease can cause an increased resistance within the portal vein leading to a build up of pressure within the portal system. This results in the development of varicose veins in the lower oesophagus (varices) which are prone to bleeding. The bleed may be severe with a mortality of up to 70%.

Key signs and symptoms
- Haematemesis
- Pale, cold, and clammy
- Restlessness and anxiety
- Altered conscious level
- Collapse

Key history and assessment
- Peptic ulcer disease
- Known liver disease
- Regular use of NSAIDs

Key observations and findings
- Pulse: <100bpm
- Cardiac monitoring is required
- BP: within normal limits
- Respiratory rate: within normal limits
- O_2 saturation: >94% on air
- Monitor and record GCS

Key investigations
- ABGs
- FBC, U&Es, glucose, LFTs, clotting factors
- Urgent cross match

Key actions and treatment
- Immediate medical support
- Maintain airway and breathing
  - ensure patent airway
  - remove blood/vomitus with a wide-bore suction catheter
  - O_2 administered via non-rebreathing mask at 15L
- Emergency anaesthetic assessment if reduced GCS or patient requiring urgent transfer to theatre
- IV access with wide-bore cannula ×2
- IV fluids and blood transfusion according to local guidelines/medical advice
- Medical/surgical referral according to local protocol
- Vasoconstrictor drug therapy (e.g. terlipressin) may be required
- Catheterization and hourly monitoring for fluid balance control.
- Provide clear explanation to patients

☼ GI bleed without cardiovascular compromise

Key signs and symptoms
- Haematemesis
- Fresh blood PR
- Melaena

Key history and assessment
- Known varices
- History of liver disease
- Repeated vomiting prior to minor haematemesis: consider Mallory–Weiss tear

Key observations and findings
- Pulse
- Cardiac monitoring is required
- BP
- Respiratory rate
- O_2 saturation

Key investigations
- FBC, U&Es, glucose, LFTs, clotting factors
- Group and save blood

Key actions and treatment
- Urgent medical review
- O_2 administered via non-rebreathing mask at 15L
- IV access with a wide-bore cannula × 2
- IV fluids
- Blood transfusion if required according to local guidelines
- Provide clear explanation to patient
- Maintain regular observations and monitoring due to risk of clinical deterioration caused by ongoing blood loss

Headache

Differential diagnosis

☼: True emergencies

- Encephalitis
- Extradural haemorrhage
- Intracerebral haemorrhage
- Meningitis
- Subarachnoid haemorrhage
- Subdural haemorrhage

✿: Urgent presentations

- Cerebral abscesses

① Timely assessment

- Cluster headache
- Migraine
- Tension-type headache

Introduction

Headache is one of the most commonly experienced health problems. The vast majority are simple self-limiting conditions which are managed by the individual without any intervention from healthcare professionals. To determine whether the patient needs further assessment to exclude serious pathology, all patients presenting with a headache require:

- Pulse
- Temperature
- Respiratory rate
- BP
- GCS

Indicators of significant underlying conditions include:

- Sudden onset
- Altered conscious level
- Fit
- Collapse
- Worst ever headache
- Significantly different from 'normal' headache
- Worse on waking
- Neck stiffness
- Abnormal vital signs
- Blackouts
- Neurological signs including visual disturbance
- Personality changes
- Hallucinations: visual or auditory

☢ Encephalitis

Encephalitis (inflammation of the brain) is usually viral in origin and can affect all age groups. Transmission may be via droplet spread, insect bites, etc. The condition is uncommon and can range in severity from a mild headache to a critical illness. Causative agents include:

- Enteroviruses
- Epstein–Barr—glandular fever
- Herpes simplex
- Influenza
- Mumps
- Polioviruses
- Rubella
- Rubeola
- Varicella

The introduction of widespread vaccination programmes has significantly reduced the incidence of encephalitis.

Bacterial encephalitis is rare and may be secondary to meningitis, sinus, or ear infections, or due to haemorrhagic spread from chest infections.

Patients with immune deficiencies are at greater risk from a wider range of infective agents. Those with HIV/AIDS can develop primary encephalitis from the HIV virus.

Key signs and symptoms
- Flu-like symptoms
- Severe headache
- Pyrexia
- N&V
- Reduced level of consciousness/confusional state
- Agitation
- Abnormal behaviour
- Sensitivity to light, photophobia
- Focal neurological signs:
  - hemiparesis
  - speech problems
  - altered sensory perception
- Focal or generalized seizures
- If encephalitis is secondary to another infection elsewhere then signs and symptoms of this infection may also be present

Key history and assessment
- Pre-existing flu-like illness
- Immunosuppression
- Recent travel to high risk areas
- Behavioural changes

Key observations and findings
- Regular recording of:
  - temperature
  - pulse

- BP
- Respiratory rate
- O_2 saturation levels
- neurological observations including GCS
- Assess patient for focal neurological deficit
- Signs of cerebral irritation—behavioural abnormalities
- Waterlow score

Key investigations

- CT brain
- Lumbar puncture: if there are no clinical or radiological signs of raised ICP
- FBC
- U&Es
- ABGs: to exclude other causes of confusion such as hypoxia, hypercarbia
- Viral titres

Key actions and treatment

- Senior medical input is urgently required
- Ensure clear airway
- Support breathing
- High-flow O_2 with non-rebreathing mask
- May require intubation and ventilation
- IV access
- IV fluids dependent on BP and blood results
- Early presentation is difficult to differentiate from meningitis therefore IV antibiotics should be given according to local guidelines
- Aciclovir IV should be given as soon as possible
- Anticonvulsants may be required
- Patients may require a darkened, quiet environment, but ensure observations can easily be carried out
- Infection control procedures should be followed
- Pressure area care if appropriate
- Patient may require admission to HDU or ICU
- In the UK encephalitis is a notifiable disease

☢ Extradural haemorrhage

📖 See Head injury, p.269.

☢ Intracerebral haemorrhage

Bleeding into the brain results in the formation of a focal haematoma which becomes a space-occupying lesion.

Causes
- Hypertension: commonest
- Anticoagulant therapy
- Vascular malformation: affects younger patients
- Bleeding disorders

Key signs and symptoms
- Dependent on the site and extent of the bleeding
- Headache
- Vomiting
- Decreased level of consciousness
- Seizures
- Focal neurological deficit

Key history and assessment
- Rapid progression of focal neurological signs
- Hypertension
- Bleeding disorders
- Anticoagulant therapy

Key observations and findings
Findings will depend on the extent and location of the bleed.
- Temperature
- Pulse
- Respiratory rate
- BP
- GCS
- Record any focal neurological deficit(s)

Key investigation
- CT brain: used to determine extent and location

Key actions and treatment
- Establish and maintain a patent airway
- Urgent referral to medical team
- Consider the need for anaesthetic assessment
- Reversal of anticoagulation if necessary, according to local protocols
- Small haematomas are usually managed conservatively
- Larger haematomas can sometimes be treated surgically

☠ Meningitis

Meningitis results from inflammation of the meningeal membranes surrounding the brain and spinal cord. The condition may be caused by viral, bacterial, or fungal infection. It affects all ages, but is more common in those aged <15 years. Viral meningitis is the most common but least severe form, rarely progressing to a serious illness. Patients with bacterial or fungal meningitis can rapidly become very ill. The speed of progression from the onset of the first signs to the development of septicaemia, collapse, and coma is one of the major challenges in management.

Causes

There are many different causative organisms including:

Viruses
- Viral meningitis:
  - Enteroviruses
  - Epstein–Barr virus

Bacteria
- *Neisseria meningitides:*
  - most common type of bacterial meningitis
  - carries a mortality rate of ~10% which increases to 20% if meningococcal septicaemia is present
- *Streptococcus pneumoniae:*
  - uncommon.
  - carries a mortality rate of 20%.
- *Tuberculosis (TB):*
  - rare
  - more common in the elderly and immunocompromised patients

Fungi
- Very rare
- Normally only found in immunocompromised patients

Key signs and symptoms

Viral meningitis
- Usually a mild self-limiting illness
- Headache
- Flu-like symptoms

Bacterial meningitis
- Fever
- Altered level of consciousness/irritability
- Severe headache
- Photophobia may be present
- Neck stiffness is an unreliable sign and is often absent
- Purpuric (non-blanching) rash indicates the presence of septicaemia

Key history and assessment
- Contact with anyone known to have recently developed meningitis
- History of flu-like symptoms
- Rapid progression of symptoms

Key observations and findings

- Airway: signs of obstruction
- Breathing:
  - tachypnoea
  - bradypnoea indicates imminent respiratory arrest, immediate anaesthetic assessment required
  - O_2 saturation, ensure levels >94%
- Circulation:
  - bradycardia due to rising intracranial pressure
  - tachycardia due to infection
  - capillary refill >2sec
  - hypotension
- Neurological observations:
  - every 30min until the patient is stable
  - if GCS falls below 15 at any time then return to every 30min
  - signs of cerebral irritation
  - focal neurological signs
  - pupils for size, equality, and reaction
- Continuous cardiac monitoring
- Pyrexia due to infection

Key investigations

- If meningococcal septicaemia is suspected treatment should not be delayed while waiting for investigations to be undertaken
- Check blood glucose
- FBC
- Blood cultures
- U&Es
- ABGs: if there are signs of septicaemia or respiratory distress
- CT scan when patient has been stabilized
- Lumbar puncture:
  - only when raised ICP has been excluded
  - to identify and isolate the organism from the CSF

Key actions and treatment

- If bacterial meningitis is suspected:
  - senior medical opinion is required immediately
  - obtain IV access: intraosseous access if unable to obtain IV
  - give antibiotics according to local/national guidelines
- O_2 via a non-rebreathing mask at 15L per min
- IV fluids
- Maintain fluid balance chart
- Pain relief
- Seizures may be controlled using anticonvulsants in accordance with local guidelines
- If patient has reduced level of consciousness:
  - immediate anaesthetics opinion
  - maintain airway
- Pressure area care
- Transfer to high dependency area or ICU
- Infection control policies should be followed at all times

- Bacterial meningitis is a notifiable disease in the UK
- Viral meningitis:
  - reassure patient
  - simple analgesia
  - conservative management

☠ Subarachnoid haemorrhage

Subarachnoid haemorrhage (SAH) is a potentially life-threatening condition which mainly affects patients aged between 35–65 years. The most common cause is a spontaneous rupture of a berry aneurysm. These small defects, which occur at the junction of an artery, are thought to be present from birth. Bleeding occurs into the space between the arachnoid and pia mater. SAH can also result from:

- Head injury
- Brain tumour

Mortality is high, with 50% of patients dying as a result of this condition.

Key signs and symptoms

- Signs and symptoms will depend on the extent of the bleed
- Headache:
  - sudden onset
  - described as like a blow to the back of the head
  - the worst headache the patient has ever experienced
- N&V may be present
- Neck stiffness may be present
- Unilateral loss of motor and/or sensory function
- Photophobia may be present
- Cerebral irritation may be present
- Altered level of consciousness
- Seizures

Key history and assessment

- Hypertension
- Up to 70% of patients have had a severe 'warning' headache in the previous 2 weeks
- Family history of cerebral aneurysm
- Illegal drug use, particularly cocaine

Key observations and findings

Findings will depend on the extent and location of the bleed:

- Temperature
- Pulse
- Respiratory rate
- BP
- GCS: the lower the GCS the worse the prognosis
- Document any focal neurological deficit

Key investigations

- CT scan:
  - as soon as airway, breathing and circulation are controlled
  - within 12 hours for all patients
  - to assess the location and extent of the bleed
- CT angiogram: to locate any vascular abnormality
- ABGs: if patient's level of consciousness is reduced
- 12-lead ECG: may show ischemic changes secondary to the SAH
- Blood glucose

Key actions and treatment

- All patients should be discussed with a neurosurgeon
- Airway management: intubation and ventilation if necessary
- IV access required
- Analgesia: morphine titrated to BP and conscious level
- If patient is conscious, oral nimodipine 60mg 4-hourly to relieve cerebral vasospasm
- If inoperable will require supportive care
- Ensure clear explanations to the patient and the family

☣ Subdural haemorrhage

📖 See Head injury, p.269

Although most commonly found as an acute condition following a severe head injury, a chronic subdural haemorrhage can occur in the days, weeks, or even months after a relatively minor head injury. The bleeding is venous in origin and results from damage to the bridging veins which run between the cortex and venous sinuses. Blood accumulates in the subdural space below the dura and above the arachnoid mater. The haematoma compresses the brain and raises the intracranial pressure. Underlying brain injury is common. The patient presents with symptoms that have progressively worsened over time.

Risk factors associated with chronic subdural haematoma include:
- Anticoagulant therapy
- Alcohol abuse
- Aged over 60 years
- Male sex

Occasionally an acute presentation can occur as the result of an arteriovenous (AV) malformation. These are most common in young men <25 years and older men >75 years.

Key signs and symptoms
- Headache
- Altered conscious level: may fluctuate with lucid periods
- Focal neurological signs:
  - hemiparesis
  - hemiplegia
  - speech defects
- Confusional state/atypical behaviour
- Personality change

Key history and assessment
- Head injury
- Anticoagulation therapy
- Gradual deterioration: chronic subdural

Key observations and findings
- Temperature
- Pulse
- BP
- Respiratory rate
- GCS
- Detailed neurological examination including pupils

Key investigation
- CT scan: to identify haematoma

Key actions and treatment
- Manage airway if patient has a reduced level of consciousness
- IV access
- Pain relief
- Refer for neurosurgical opinion
- Give sufficient IV fluids to maintain adequate BP and cerebral perfusion pressure

:⚕: **Cerebral abscess**

Cerebral abscess refers to a collection of pus within the brain. Causes include:
- Ear infections
- Sinus infections
- Compound skull fracture
- Intracranial surgery
- Dental infections
- Pulmonary infections

Key signs and symptoms
- Headache
- Pyrexia
- N&V
- Altered GCS may be present
- Focal neurological signs
- Seizure

Key history and assessment
- History of flu-like symptoms
- Recent infection especially otitis media or sinusitis
- Recent dental work
- Any changes in behaviour or personality?

Key observations and findings
- Ensure clear airway
- Observe breathing
- Monitor O_2 saturation: ensure levels not <94%
- Pulse and BP
- Regular neurological observations: document any focal deficit
- Temperature

Key investigations
- FBC, U&Es
- CT scan: to confirm diagnosis and help locate the position of the abscess
- Blood cultures if patient febrile

Key actions and treatment
- Establish and maintain a patent airway if depressed conscious level: if any compromise call for anaesthetic opinion
- High-dose O_2 15L via a non-rebreathing mask
- Cardiac monitoring
- IV access required
- Treat seizures according to local guidelines
- Early use of antibiotics: obtain expert advice
- Urgent referral to neurosurgery as drainage of abscess is likely to be required
- Provide analgesia
- Protect patient from injury due to disorientation
- Reassure at all times and explain procedures whether or not you think they understand
- If unconscious, maintain strict pressure area care for skin integrity

ⓘ Cluster headache

Cluster headaches are relatively rare, affecting <1 in 1000 people. The cause is unknown but they are thought to be related to migraine.

Key signs and symptoms

- Severe unilateral pain
- Short lasting, often <1 hour
- Clustered in groups:
  - several attacks a day for a number of weeks
  - gap of months or years before another cluster of attacks occurs
- Pain centered around one eye
- Inflammation and watering to eye
- Nasal congestion on same side as pain

Key history and assessment

- Sudden onset
- Look for triggers such as:
  - alcohol
  - strong smells such as solvents, strong perfumes, petrol
  - extreme heat
- Pain at the same time each day
- Often woken by pain during the night, within 2 hours of going to sleep
- Sometimes woken by pain in the early morning
- 80% of patients are male

Key observations and findings

- Ensure no focal neurological signs
- Pulse
- Temperature: to exclude infection
- Respiratory rate
- BP

Key investigations

- If there is any suspicion of SAH, for example, first presentation, then investigate as for SAH
- None in emergency care
- Primary care may refer to neurologist for investigation

Key actions and treatment

- Simple analgesia
- Darkened room
- Quiet environment
- Migraine treatment: sumatriptan 100mg orally or 6mg SC may be used

⊕ Migraine

A recurrent debilitating headache which has consistent features for each individual patient. Symptoms may last up to 3 days.

Key signs and symptoms

The diagnosis of migraine requires two of the following symptoms:
- Unilateral pain
- Throbbing pain
- Worse on movement
- Moderate or severe pain which stops people functioning normally

Plus one of the following symptoms:
- Nausea or vomiting
- Sensitivity to light—photophobia
- Sensitivity to sounds—phonophobia

Other signs and symptoms include:
- Preceding aura
- Abdominal pain
- Visual disturbances
- Focal neurological signs

Key history and assessment

- First onset in late teens or early 20s
- Family history of close relative with migraine
- Pain worse on movement
- Aura immediately before the attack:
  - flashing lights
  - smells
  - pins and needles
- Trigger factors:
  - menstrual cycles
  - coffee
  - cheese
  - chocolate
  - oral contraceptive pill
  - over–tired
  - red wine
  - monosodium glutamate.
- Periods of stress or anxiety

Key observations and findings

- Pulse
- Respiratory rate
- BP
- Temperature

Key investigations

- None normally required

Key actions and treatment
- Anti-emetic: metoclopramide
- Simple analgesia:
  - taken early may lessen severity
  - aspirin
  - paracetamol
  - codeine effervescent for quick action
- Darkened room and quiet environment
- Sumatriptan 100mg orally or 6mg SC may be used

① Tension-type headache

The most common type of headache whose exact aetiology is still unknown, despite it being one of the most frequently experienced disorders. Up to 90% of women and 70% of men are believed to suffer from tension-type headaches, with the peak incidence being between the ages of 20–50 years.

Key signs and symptoms
- Pain:
  - mild-to-moderate pain
  - described as tightness or pressure
  - dull ache
  - across the forehead
  - base of skull/ top of the neck
- Tightness or ache across shoulders
- No nausea
- May last minutes or days

Key history and assessment
- Is this headache different than those which the patient normally experiences?
- Has the patient taken any analgesics and have they been effective?
- Symptoms which may require further assessment include:
  - sudden onset of severe pain
  - accompanying pyrexia
  - rash
  - focal neurological signs
  - onset of new headache pain after age 50
  - recent head injury

Key observations and findings
- Temperature
- Document any focal neurological deficit

Key investigations
- None required

Key actions and treatment
- Simple analgesia:
  - what suits the patient?
  - what has worked before?
  - NSAIDs as a first choice
  - paracetamol if patient can't take NSAIDs
- Patient should be reassured that the condition is self-limiting

Further reading

Royal College of Physicians Clinical Effectiveness and Evaluation Unit (2004). *National Clinical Guidelines for Stroke*, 2nd edition. London: Royal College of Physicians.

Head injury

Differential diagnosis

⚙ Urgent presentations
- Significant head injury

ⓘ Timely assessment
- Scalp lacerations and haematoma
- Minor head injury

Introduction

Head injuries are common and range in severity from minor to life-threatening. Primary brain injury occurs at the time of the initial trauma. Secondary injuries occur due to subsequent intracranial bleeding, hypoxia, or inadequate cerebral perfusion. As for all trauma patients initial management should focus on maintaining airway, breathing, and circulation. The exact nature of the head injury should be ascertained as part of the secondary survey.

Raised intracranial pressure (ICP)

Intracranial bleeding or cerebral swelling will increase the pressure within the skull which is a potentially life-threatening condition. Be aware that the signs of raised ICP (hypertension and bradycardia) may mask the signs of hypovolaemia.

Intracranial bleeding

Intracranial haemorrhage is the commonest reason for surgical intervention following head injury.

Extradural haemorrhage

An extradural haemorrhage is an accumulation of blood between the dura and skull which may result from a fracture of the temporal or parietal bone. Bleeding occurs from the middle meningeal vessels. As the haematoma develops the brain is compressed and the ICP rises. This is a neurosurgical emergency, requiring urgent referral. Successful drainage of the haematoma often results in a good long-term outcome for the patient.

Subdural haemorrhage

A subdural haemorrhage results from shearing of the bridging veins which run between the cortex and venous sinuses. Blood accumulates in the subdural space below the dura and above the arachnoid membrane. The haematoma may compress the brain and raise the ICP. Associated cerebral injury is very common; as a result a full neurological recovery is less likely than for an isolated extradural haemorrhage. Signs and symptoms of subdural haemorrhage may sometimes be delayed for days or weeks (chronic subdural) as venous bleeding occurs more slowly than arterial bleeds. Once the patient has been stabilized urgent neurosurgical advice is necessary.

Traumatic SAH

SAH following a severe head injury is caused by bleeding of the cerebral vessels into the space between the arachnoid and pia mater. Again, urgent neurosurgical advice is required following stabilization of the patient.

Intracerebral haemorrhage and contusion

Shearing forces resulting from trauma can cause tearing of vessels within the brain leading to an intracerebral haemorrhage. Bruising within the brain (cerebral contusions) occurs as a result of coup (below site of impact) or contra-coup (opposite the site of impact) injuries as the brain strikes the skull. These injuries do not usually require emergency neurosurgical intervention. However neurosurgical advice should be sought.

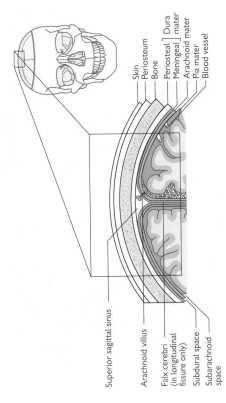

Skin
Periosteum
Bone
Periosteal ⎤ Dura
Meningeal ⎦ mater
Arachnoid mater
Pia mater
Blood vessel

Superior sagittal sinus

Arachnoid villus

Falx cerebri
(in longitudinal
fissure only)

Subdural space

Subarachnoid
space

Fig. 25.1 Meninges.

Neurological observations

Level of consciousness

The patients level of consciousness (LOC) can be assessed using the AVPU scale or the GCS.

AVPU

The mnemonic AVPU is a quick and consistent method of assessing conscious level often used by ambulance personnel and other front line health professionals.

- **A**: **A**lert
- **V**: responds to **V**oice
- **P**: responds to **P**ain
- **U**: **U**nresponsive

It is recorded by highlighting the appropriate letter from the mnemonic.

Glasgow Coma Score (GCS)

The GCS is a more detailed assessment tool for recording and monitoring a patient's LOC. A GCS of <15 is considered an altered conscious level. A score of 9–13 is a significant reduction, and patients with a score of 8 or less are considered to be in coma. The GCS allows assessment of overall cerebral function by recording a patient's physiological response to stimuli in three areas:

- Eye opening
- Verbal response
- Motor responses

Each component is scored separately and the results added together. For example a fully alert patient would score: E4 V5 M6 = GCS 15

Eye opening (scored out of 4)

- 4. Spontaneous: the patient's eyes are open
- 3. To speech: the patient's eyes only open after being spoken to:
  - be aware of patients with hearing problems
  - be aware of patients who may not speak English
- 2. To pain: physical stimulation is required to obtain an eye opening response—firm pressure on the supra orbital ridge
- 1. No eye opening:
  - observe for orbital swelling which may prevent eye opening
  - if the eyelids are swollen shut then the letter C should be used for closed rather than depicting a score for no eye opening

Verbal response (scored out of 5)

Ask the patient clear simple questions which they should be able to answer, e.g. Can you tell me what day it is? Can you tell me which town you are in?

- 5. Orientated: patient responds fully to the questions asked
- 4. Confused: patient answers incorrectly to simple questions (e.g. time, person, place)
- 3. Inappropriate: gives answers out of context to the questioned asked
- 2. Incomprehensible: no recognizable words/incomprehensible sounds
- 1. No response: patient makes no sounds at all

If the patient is intubated or has a tracheostomy the letter T should be used for tubed rather than depicting a score for no response.

Motor response (scored out of 6)

Ask the patient to perform simple and direct movements. Such as, can you lift your right arm?

- 6. Obeys commands: patient understands and performs requested movement
- 5. Localization to pain: patient does not respond to commands but responds to a painful stimulus by trying to remove the source of the pain, i.e. tries to locate and push away the hand or finger at the pressure point
- 4. Flexion withdrawal: patient responds to painful stimuli by flexing arms at elbows
- 3. Abnormal flexion: patient responds to painful stimuli by flexing arms at elbow but pronating arms and making a fist whilst plantar flexing feet (decorticate rigidity)
- 2. Abnormal extension: patient responds to stimuli by straightening elbows and abducting arms whilst internally rotating and palms pronated to pain (decerebrate rigidity)
- 1. No response: patient does not respond to painful stimuli and no change in tone of limb is observed

In addition to level of consciousness pupillary reaction and limb movement/ tone should be assessed and recorded.

Pupillary assessment

Pupils are examined for size, shape, and reaction to light. The pupils should be round and equal in size, constricting in response to light.

Limb movements

Abnormal limb movement or muscle tone may indicate focal neurological problems. Ask the patient to perform simple movements and compare both sides.

- Normal power: patient can move limbs according to normal muscle tone
- Mild weakness: patient can move one limb showing normal strength but the opposite is weaker
- Severe weakness: patient shows marked difference between the two limbs
- No movement: patient has no response against painful stimuli

Neurological observation should be charted clearly so that no ambiguity can occur in interpretation (Fig. 25.2).

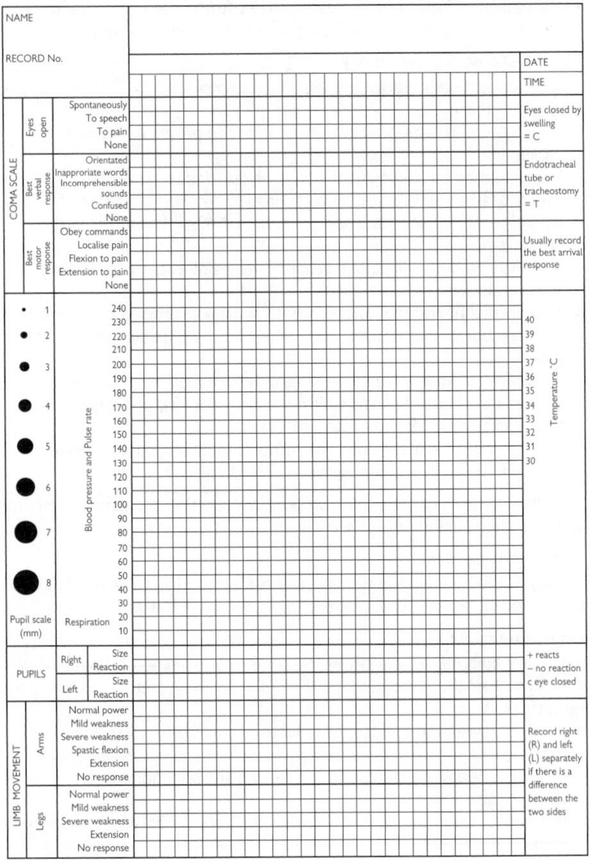

Fig. 25.2 Neurological observations chart

☼ Significant head injury

Key signs and symptoms
- GCS <15
- Focal neurological deficit:
  - pupillary abnormalities: dilation, irregular, fixed
  - abnormal speech
  - muscle weakness
  - decreased sensation
  - abnormal reflexes
- Suspicion of skull fracture:
  - visible trauma to head
  - CSF from ears/nose
  - bleeding from ear
  - black eye with no associated local trauma
  - bruising behind ear on mastoid process: Battle's sign
- Seizures
- Vomiting, may be projectile
- Pre- or post-traumatic amnesia
- Persistent headache

Key history and assessment
- High energy mechanism of injury:
  - pedestrian hit by a motor vehicle
  - occupant thrown from a motor vehicle
  - fall from a height of >1m or 5 stairs
  - diving incident
  - high speed road traffic collision
  - rollover motor incident
  - incident involving motorized recreational vehicle
  - bicycle collision
- Any reported loss of consciousness
- Previous neurosurgery
- Drug or alcohol intoxication
- Anticoagulant therapy: warfarin
- Age 65 or older
- Altered behaviour
- Wounds:
  - position, site, shape, and edges
  - FBs/dirt
  - underlying structures—vessels, bone
  - 'boggy' area on the scalp

Any patient presenting with any of the these findings will require further medical assessment and management

Key observations and findings
- Respirations: rate and effectiveness
- Pulse: tachycardia may indicate haemorrhage from other injuries
- BP: hypotension may indicate haemorrhage from other injuries
- GCS: should be recorded every 30min initially

- Pupillary response
- Limb power and movement
- O$_2$ saturation
- Temperature: hypothermia may result from prolonged exposure

Accurate recording and interpretation of neurological indicators and vital signs are essential when caring for patients with head injuries. They should be recorded every 30min in patients with a GCS of <15 until their conscious level returns to normal. For patients with a GCS of 15 who require observation, this should be undertaken every 30min for the first 2 hours, then hourly for the next 4 hours and 2-hourly after this until discontinued. If at any time the GCS falls, obtain urgent medical advice and return the interval between observations to 30min.

Key investigations
- Blood specimens:
  - ABGs: if any signs of respiratory distress or hypoxia
  - FBC
  - blood glucose
  - U&Es
  - group and save/cross match according to the condition of the patient
- CT is the recommended investigation for patients with a significant head injury. Skull XR is no longer considered to be appropriate[1]

Key indicators for CT within the hour
- GCS <13 at any time since the injury
- GCS = 13 or 14 at 2 hours after the injury
- Focal neurological deficit
- Suspected open or depressed skull fracture
- Signs of basal skull fracture:
  - haemotympanum
  - panda eyes
  - CSF otorrhoea
  - bruising of the mastoid process: Battle's sign
- Post-traumatic seizure
- > 1 episode of vomiting
- Amnesia for >30min post-injury

In addition, a CT within an hour should be considered if any of the following features are present:
- Loss of consciousness or amnesia
- >65 years
- Coagulopathy:
  - history of bleeding
  - clotting disorder
  - warfarin therapy

Alternatively, the presence of any of the following features should trigger a CT scan within 8 hours of the injury:
- Dangerous mechanism:
  - pedestrian struck by a motor vehicle
  - occupant ejected from a motor vehicle
  - fall from a height of >1m or 5 stairs

- Amnesia of >30min before the incident

All patients with a significant head injury should be considered at risk for a cervical spine injury and XRs or CT will be required following assessment by an experienced clinician.

Key actions and treatments

Initial treatment should follow the principles of trauma management:

- Airway:
  - call for anaesthetic opinion if airway compromise is present
  - consider the potential for a cervical spine injury when maintaining a patient's airway
- Breathing: high-flow O_2 15L via non-rebreathing mask
- Circulation:
  - IV access required, 2 × large-bore IV cannulae
  - IV fluids as required
  - maintain fluid balance chart
  - pressure dressings for significant bleeding points
- Disability: fits may be controlled using anticonvulsants
- Environment:
  - protect patient from further injury where possible
  - maintain pressure area care for skin integrity
  - ensure no loss of body heat
- Pain relief: IV analgesia titrated to the patient's response
- Explain procedures to patient whether or not you think he/she understands

Referral to neurosurgery

- New surgically significant abnormalities on imaging
- Persistent coma GCS <8
- Unexplained confusion for >4 hours
- Deterioration in GCS
- Progressive focal signs
- Seizure without full recovery
- Penetrating injury
- CSF leak

Transfer to neurological centre

- Consultant to consultant referral for transfer
- Resuscitation and stabilization should be completed before transfer

Criteria for admission

- New clinically significant abnormalities on imaging
- GCS <15
- Patients who require CT which cannot be undertaken for whatever reason
- Persistent vomiting
- Severe headache
- Drug or alcohol intoxication
- History of seizure
- Other injuries
- CSF leak

Criteria for discharge

- GCS must be 15
- Significant injuries must be ruled out prior to discharge
- Only if the risk of late complications is minimal should a patient with a significant mechanism of injury be discharged without suitable supervision arrangements in place
- If the patient is to be discharged, written head-injury instructions should be given

Further reading

1. National Institute for Clinical Excellence (2007). *Head Injury. Triage, assessment, investigation and early management of head injury in infants, children and adults.* London: NICE.

⚠ Scalp lacerations and haematoma

The patient's scalp needs careful examination to assist in excluding a penetrating head injury, an underlying skull fracture, and the possibility of a significant head injury. Head wounds which bleed extensively can be extremely frightening for patients and relatives.

Key signs and symptoms
- Obvious wound
- Boggy swelling
- Obvious bleeding

Key history and assessment
- Mechanism of injury
- Pre-existing medical condition
- Anticoagulant therapy

Key observations and findings
- GCS: should be 15
- Neurological observations: should be normal
- Vital signs: should be normal
- Extent of haemorrhage

Key investigations
- None usually required

Key actions and treatments
- Attempt to control bleeding with direct pressure
- Wounds should be fully explored and cleaned prior to closure
- Simple linear wounds can be closed with sutures or staples
- Deep wounds need to be closed in layers to prevent further bleeding and haematoma formation
- Complex wounds may require a GA and exploration and closure in theatre
- Written head injury instructions and wound care advice should be provided

① **Minor head injury**

A diagnosis of minor head injury can be made if the patient meets the following criteria:
- Transient or no loss of consciousness at scene
- No seizures
- GCS 15
- No focal neurological deficit
- Minor mechanism of injury
- No other significant injuries

The patient can be considered for discharge if a responsible adult is present and verbal and written head injury advice are provided.

Limb problems

Differential diagnosis

☺ True emergencies
- Amputation
- Arterial embolism
- Compartment syndrome
- Haemorrhage
- Myocardial infarction

☼ Urgent presentations
- Deep vein thrombosis
- Musculoskeletal injury

① Timely assessment
- Infection
- Inflammatory disorders

☠ Amputation

Any limb can be affected at any level with the amputation being partial or complete. The mechanism of injury will be crushing, avulsion, or guillotining. Clean guillotine injuries are the most likely to be successful in reattachment. If the damaged part is still partially attached it should be supported and splinted, with pressure applied to any bleeding. If the amputation is complete the severed part should be wrapped in a clean dressing and placed in a cold container. If ice is used the limb must not come into contact with it as further tissue damage can occur. A clean towel, cloth, or layer of plastic should be used to protect the part. Direct pressure should be applied to the remaining limb to restrict the bleeding.

☠ Arterial embolism

An embolus, often originating from the heart, may obstruct an artery resulting in peripheral ischaemia. If blood flow is not restored rapidly, irreversible tissue damage may occur which can threaten the viability of the limb.

Key signs and symptoms

The effects of acute embolism are classically described as the 6 Ps:
- **P**ain: usually severe
- **P**ulseless: distal to the embolism
- **P**allor: pale skin colour
- **P**erishing cold: both to the patient and on touch
- **P**araesthesia: altered sensation, pins and needles, tingling
- **P**aralysis: as a result of nerve and muscle ischaemia

Key history and assessment

- Atrial fibrillation
- Recent MI
- Mitral stenosis
- Aortic aneurysm
- Recent trauma

Key observations and findings

- Absent or weak distal pulse
- Pale/cool distal limb
- Decreased or absent BP distal to occlusion
- Respiratory rate should be normal, may be increased due to pain

Key investigations

- Doppler ultrasound, 12-lead ECG
- FBC, U&E, blood glucose, group and save
- Angiography

Key actions and treatment

- Urgent medical review
- Pain relief, normally IV
- IV fluids

☠ Compartment syndrome

Increased pressure within the fascial compartments of the limbs can occur as a result of trauma. A direct blow, with or without a fracture, or a muscle tear can cause haemorrhage and/or tissue swelling. Overuse as a result of prolonged physical exercise may also cause considerable tissue swelling. In addition prolonged localized pressure (an unconscious patient having prolonged surgery or a plaster of Paris) can lead to significant tissue oedema resulting in compartment syndrome. In a number of cases no obvious cause is found.

The tough fascia surrounding the muscle compartments cannot stretch to accommodate the swelling. As a consequence the compartment pressure rises, eventually becoming sufficiently high to cause compression of capillaries. This causes ischaemia which results in further swelling, compounding the problem. Following the initial injury, symptoms develop between 2 hours and 6 days. If compartment syndrome is not identified and treated promptly, irreversible damage to muscles and nerves will result. Muscle cell breakdown results in release of potassium and myogloblin which can cause cardiac arrhythmias and renal failure respectively.

Key signs and symptoms
- Severe pain: disproportionate to apparent injury
- Pain exacerbated by passive muscle stretching or palpation
- Paraesthesia
- Reduced motor function due to pain or neurological dysfunction
- Pale/cool limb

Key history and assessment
- Recent history of injury especially:
  - crush injury
  - burns
  - fractures
  - splintage
- Prolonged localized pressure:
  - unconscious patients
  - immobile patients
  - recent surgery

Key observations and findings
- *Distal pulses may be present at first*
- *Pulselessness is a late sign*

Key investigations
- Diagnosis should be made clinically
- U&E: this will assist in early detection of hyperkalaemia
- ABGs
- Urinalysis: to look for myoglobinuria

Key actions and treatment
- Cardiac monitoring
- Remove plaster of Paris, splints, dressings or bandages

- Obtain urgent medical review
- IV access and fluid to maintain normal BP
- Elevate limb
- Analgesia as appropriate to pain, may require IV analgesia
- Treat cardiac arrhythmias, if present, according to ALS guidelines

☠ Haemorrhage

Haemorrhage from the limbs can range from superficial lacerations to life-threatening bleeds from arterial injuries. It is important to recognize that bleeding may be occult (e.g. following fracture of a long bone).

The most serious complication of haemorrhage is hypovolaemic shock, which results in inadequate tissue perfusion. Hypovolaemia resulting from haemorrhage may be classified into 4 groups as follows:

- Class I: up to 750mL, 15% of blood volume
- Class II: up to 1500mL, 15–30% of blood volume
- Class III: up to 2000mL, 30–40% of blood volume
- Class IV: over 2500mL, 40% of blood volume

Key signs and symptoms
- Type of bleeding:
  - pulsating, bright red—arterial
  - steady flow, dull red—venous
  - ooze—capillary
- Obvious deformity and swelling suggesting long bone fracture

Key history and assessment
- Mechanism of injury
- Time of injury
- Extent of injury
- Estimated amount of blood loss
- Current medications, especially anticoagulants
- Pre-existing medical conditions

Key observations and findings
- Class I:
  - mild tachycardia
  - no change in respiratory rate
  - no change in BP
- Class II:
  - increased respiratory rate
  - cool, clammy skin
  - tachycardia
  - thirst
- Class III:
  - tachypnoea
  - tachycardia
  - reduced BP
  - confusion/aggression
  - oliguria
- Class IV:
  - tachypnoea or bradypnoea: peri-arrest
  - tachycardia
  - decreased or unrecordable BP
  - impalpable peripheral pulses
  - cold, pale skin
  - reduced level of consciousness
  - anuria

Key investigations
- Class II and above:
  - FBC, U&Es, ABGs
  - blood glucose
  - group and save/cross match blood as appropriate

Key actions and treatment
- Ensure personal protection by the use of gloves, gown, and eye protection
- Commence cardiac, BP, SpO_2 monitoring
- Minor haemorrhage:
  - elevate the limb if possible
  - remove any obvious dirt or debris
  - apply direct pressure to the bleeding until stopped
  - clean, close, and dress wound as appropriate
  - assess need for anti-tetanus cover and antibiotic cover—see local guidelines
- Major haemorrhage:
  - obtain urgent medical assistance
  - lie the patient down with the head lower than the body
  - elevate the limb if possible
  - high-flow O_2 via a non-rebreathing mask
  - insert 2 short large-bore cannula, in the antecubital fossa if possible
  - commence fluid replacement
  - consider the need for transfusion
  - monitor urine output
  - do not remove any embedded FBs
  - apply direct pressure to the bleeding using gauze or other suitable dressing or pad
  - if bleeding continues through dressing, do not remove, add another on top
  - if obvious major arterial bleeding apply indirect pressure to the proximal artery

☠ Myocardial infarction

The presence of pain in the left arm is well recognized as an indicator of MI. Although it is often secondary to central chest pain it can, on occasion, present alone. It should always be considered if no other reason for the limb problem is found.

📖 See Chest pain, p.115.

☢ Deep vein thrombosis

The term DVT describes the formation of a thrombus in the deep veins of the limbs. Many small DVTs are asymptomatic. However, potentially fatal pulmonary embolus can occur if the thrombus becomes detached and obstructs the pulmonary vessels.

Key signs and symptoms
- Swelling distal to the thrombus
- Redness and warmth of the distal limb
- Dull aching pain, worse on standing or walking
- Usually, though not always, affects only one limb

Key history and assessment
- Up to 95% of people with DVT will have at least one of the following aspects in their history:
  - 40+ age group are at greater risk
  - previous history of DVT
  - family history of DVT
  - treatment for cancer within the previous 6 months
  - heart failure and circulation problems
  - recent surgery, especially hip or knee
  - pregnant women or recent childbirth
  - combined contraceptive pill
  - hormone replacement therapy
- Smoking may increase the risk of DVT
- Long-haul flights are increasingly being seen as a risk factor
- Prolonged immobilization
- Obesity

The Wells score is a tool commonly used to determine the level of probability of DVT[1]. Criteria are assessed as shown in Table 26.1.

Table 26.1 Wells score

Clinical characteristic	Score
Active cancer: treatment ongoing, administered within previous 6 months or palliative	1
Paralysis, paresis or recent plaster immobilization of the lower extremities	1
Recently bedridden >3 days or major surgery within previous 12 weeks requiring general or regional anaesthesia	1
Localized tenderness along the distribution of the deep venous system	1
Swelling of entire leg	1
Calf swelling >3cm larger than asymptomatic side—measured 10cm below tibial tuberosity	1
Pitting oedema confined to symptomatic leg	1
Collateral superficial veins—nonvaricose	1
Previously documented DVT	1
Alternative diagnosis at least as likely as DVT	−2

A score of ≥2 indicates that the probability of DVT is likely. A score of <2 indicates that the probability is unlikely.

Key observations and findings
- Mild pyrexia due to inflammatory response
- The presence of tachycardia, dyspnoea, low BP, or pleuritic chest pain should raise suspicion of a pulmonary embolism

Key investigations
- D-dimer: if Wells score indicates low probability
- Doppler ultrasound
- Venogram

Key actions and treatment
- Check for signs and symptoms of pulmonary embolism,
  📖 see Pulmonary embolism, p.128.
- Low molecular weight heparin according to local guidelines
- Compression stockings reduce the risk of developing post-thrombotic syndrome
- Follow-up in primary care or specialist DVT service: see local guidelines

:❂: Musculoskeletal injuries

Musculoskeletal injuries only become true emergencies when major haemorrhage or acute neurological damage is present. All patients should be assessed in order to exclude serious injury and to facilitate adequate pain control. Some musculoskeletal injuries may appear dramatic, but they should not distract the healthcare professional from undertaking assessment and management of airway, breathing, and circulation.

Key signs and symptoms

- Compound (open) fracture:
  - any break in skin integrity combined with an underlying fracture
  - significant risk of infection
- Critical skin:
  - gross deformity of a limb may stretch the skin, compromising cutaneous circulation
  - risk of injury becoming open as ischemic skin becomes necrotic
- Gross deformity:
  - indicates significant musculoskeletal injury
  - severe pain
  - risk of critical skin
  - risk of neurovascular injury
- Neurological deficit:
  - altered sensation
  - often associated with vascular injury
- Loss of function or reduction in the range of movement in a limb

Key history and assessment

- History of trauma
- Mechanism of injury
- Predisposing relevant medical conditions—e.g. osteoporosis
- Consider associated injuries
- Apply validated assessment tools if appropriate
  - Ottawa ankle rules[2]
  - Ottawa knee rule[3]
- Pain scoring
- Normal level of mobility for patient
- Social circumstances: particularly important in the elderly

Key observations and findings

- Distal pulses
- Distal sensation
- Active movement
- Passive movement
- Power: compare with other limb.
- Balanced skin overlying deformity indicates threatened cutaneous circulation

Key investigations

- XR of the area(s) if indicated
- Ankle dislocations can result in neurovascular compromise. If this is evident then reduction should occur prior to XR

Key actions and treatment

- Pain relief:
  - nitrous oxide/O_2 (Entonox®)
  - IV/oral analgesia as appropriate
  - immobilize with splint or sling as appropriate
- Open fractures:
  - minimize blood loss
  - apply sterile dressing reduce risk of infection
  - IV antibiotics—see local guidelines
  - urgent referral to orthopaedics
- Closed fracture:
  - arrange for definitive treatment according to local guidelines
  - refer to orthopaedics if admission is required
  - fracture clinic follow-up if patient is fit for discharge
- Dislocation:
  - exclude associated fracture
  - medical review for relocation as soon as possible
  - discharge or admit as appropriate
- Isolated soft tissue injury
  - dressing and closure of wounds as appropriate
  - advice regarding mobilization, elevation and simple analgesia as required.
  - physiotherapy may be helpful

Further reading

1. Scarvelis D and Wells PS (2006). Diagnosis and treatment of deep-vein thrombosis. *CMAJ*, **175**, 1087–92.
2. Stiell IG, McKnight RD, Greenberg GH, *et al.* (1994). Implementation of the Ottawa ankle rules. *JAMA*, **271**, 827–32.
3. Stiell IG, Wells GA, Hoag RH, *et al.* (1997) Implementation of the Ottawa knee rule for the use of radiography in acute knee injuries. *JAMA*, **278**, 2075–9.

① **Inflammatory disorders**

A wide range of inflammatory disorders can affect the limbs. Most are managed in the primary care setting. However, a few conditions may present to the emergency department/MIU. These include:
• Olecranon/patellar bursitis
• Gout

Bursitis

Bursitis presents as a localized swelling over the extensor surface of the elbow or knee. The swelling is often significant and disproportionate to the pain which may be present. Joint movement is not painful although it may be restricted by the swelling. This condition should not be confused with septic arthritis, where joint movement is extremely painful and the patient is often systemically unwell. Treatment of bursitis usually involves NSAIDs.

Gout

Gout is an inflammatory condition which predominantly affects the joints of the big toe and knee. The patient presents with severe pain and an obvious swelling over the affected joint which has a shiny, red appearance. Pain is worsened by movement and the patient may feel unwell. The condition is associated with the use of certain medications (such as diuretics), renal failure, etc. Obtain medical advice prior to treatment.

① **Infection**

A wide range of infections can affect the limbs. Most limb infections are minor and will resolve with oral antibiotics. However, osteomyelitis and septic arthritis are serious condition which require urgent assessment and intervention.

📖 See Abscesses and local infection, p.19.

Major trauma

Differential diagnosis

☼ True emergencies

- Primary survey and resuscitation
- Secondary survey
- Definitive treatment

Introduction

In patients under the age of 45, major trauma is the most common cause of death in developed counties and second only to HIV/AIDS worldwide. It can be defined as the consequences of an incident which results in potentially life or limb-threatening injuries. The majority of people who die following a major trauma will do so at the scene. If the patient survives the immediate trauma, haemorrhage is the principal cause of death.

Over the last 25 years guidelines and protocols have been developed and adopted around the world based on a systematic approach to trauma care. These principles are taught though programmes such as Trauma Nursing Core Courses (TNCC), Advanced Trauma Life Support (ATLS), and Pre-Hospital Trauma Life Support (PHTLS). Staff working in an area likely to receive patients with major trauma should receive appropriate training.

There are 4 main stages to the management of major trauma:
• Safety
• Primary survey
• Secondary survey
• Definitive care

Each must be addressed and managed prior to moving on to the next stage. All assessments should take into account the mechanism of injury and the resulting potential patterns of injury.

Safety

The safety of the environment must be assessed to prevent further harm occurring either to the patient, healthcare professionals, or bystanders.

The following questions should be asked:
• Is it safe to approach the patient?
• What is required to make the environment safe?
• Will the area remain safe?
• Is anyone else present who can help?
• Who is taking the lead in managing the patient?
• Is help required?
• If so from whom?
• If there is more than one victim who should to be assessed first?
• Does the patient need to be moved, and how can this be achieved?

:☠: Primary survey and resuscitation

The primary survey is aimed at the identification and management of immediately life-threatening problems and is based on the assessment of ABCDE. Any problem found should be corrected before moving further on in the assessment. If the patient's condition deteriorates at any stage then the primary survey should be repeated.

Airway with cervical spine control

- Protect the cervical spine
- Hold the head in alignment with the body
- A second person should apply a semi-rigid cervical collar
- Immobilize head with sandbags or blocks
- Prevent neck movement by placing tape across the forehead and under the chin, anchoring each to the trolley
- Ensure you are in the patient's eyeline when speaking
- Ensure patient is aware they should not move their head
- Ensure the airway is patent—jaw thrust may be required
- Suction should be available with a rigid tonsil tip catheter—Yankeur
- Airway intervention may be required:
  - nasopharyngeal airway—can be used in conscious patients who do not have facial or head trauma
  - oropharyngeal airway—only for use in unresponsive patients
  - intubation—experienced practitioner required, secures airway from inhalation

Breathing

- High-flow O_2 via non-rebreathing mask should be used initially
- Observe chest movements, tracheal position
- Listen for breath sounds, feel for exhaled breath if necessary
- Assess rate, effort, and adequacy of breathing
- Signs of hypoxia: altered conscious level, confusion, aggression
- SpO_2 measurement
- Ventilation can be assisted with a bag/valve/mask device: this is a two-person technique
- Check for chest wounds
- Breathing should be frequently reassessed

Circulation and haemorrhage control

- Pulse: rate, rhythm, quality
- Cardiac resuscitation if no pulse present—extremely poor prognosis
- Capillary refill assessment: should normally be <2sec
- Signs of hypovolaemia: tachycardia, decreased BP, altered conscious level
- External haemorrhage requires direct pressure or elevation
- IV access, 2 × wide-bore cannula
- Intraosseous access may be needed or IV venous cut down
- IV fluid according to local policy
- Blood for group and save/cross match as required: may need type specific or O negative if severe bleeding
- ECG monitoring

- BP monitoring
- Any penetrating objects must be left in situ

Disability, dysfunction
- Assess neurological state using AVPU:
  - A: **a**lert
  - V: responding to **voice**
  - P: responds to **pain**
  - U: **u**nresponsive
- Record GCS, regularly: every 30min initially
- Assess pupil size and reaction
- Assess limb power and reflexes if possible
- Consider possible reversible causes:
  - hypoxia
  - hypoglycemia
  - substance misuse

Exposure/environmental control
- Check and maintain patient's temperature
  - warm room
  - warm IV fluids
  - warm blankets
  - warming devices—bair hugger
- Fully exposure patient to examine: recover afterwards to prevent hypothermia
- Log roll

☣: Secondary survey

The purpose of the secondary survey is to identify other significant injuries. The assessment should be from head to toe and progress in an orderly manner with all findings, both positive and negative, recorded. Major problems such as an unstable pelvic fracture may require immediate treatment in order to reduce haemorrhage. Other injuries may require specialist assessment and treatment.

☣: Definitive treatment

Definitive treatment will depend upon injuries found during the primary and secondary surveys. The appropriate specialist(s) should be involved. If the patient is to be transferred, clear arrangements must be in place with the name of the accepting doctor and team confirmed, the location to which the patient is to be transferred agreed, and the necessary equipment and skilled staff available for the transfer. All documentation must be complete and taken with the patient. As far as possible the patient should be stabilized prior to transfer. If the patient remains unstable with ongoing bleeding then transfer directly to theatre as quickly as possible to facilitate haemostasis.

Mental health

Differential diagnosis

☼ Urgent presentations

- Aggression
- Hypomania/mania
- Perceptual disorders (psychoses)

① Timely assessment

- Panic disorder
- Self-harm

② Non-urgent presentations

- Eating disorders

Mental health

Mental health emergencies can be frightening and challenging for both patients and staff. They can be defined as acute disturbances of thought, mood, or behaviour which may result in to harm to the patient or others. Possible organic causes need to be identified and the extent to which they are contributing to the patient's presentation should be determined.

:۞: Aggression

Relatively few aggressive or violent incidents occur as a direct result of mental health problems. Most commonly aggression results from alcohol intoxication or substance misuse. Most aggressive incidents are preceded by a number of warning signs and staff should recognize these and act to defuse situations if they can do so without placing themselves at risk. The presence of security staff or police may be required for staff and patient safety. It is important to exclude reversible causes (e.g. hypoglycemia) and to identify serious conditions such as head injury.

📖 See Behaving strangely, p.75.

☼ Hypomania/mania

Hypomania and mania are components of bipolar affective disorder (sometimes referred to as manic depression). Hypomania describes the presence of an elevated mood, high levels of energy, high self-esteem, self-confidence, and unfounded optimism which is maintained regardless of circumstances. There is a loss of insight. Patients can present as an emergency when their behaviour starts to affect those around them and interferes with their ability to function. This is particularly the case with mania where the symptoms are particularly severe. Psychotic symptoms such as paranoia may occur where the patient loses touch with reality and can become a danger to themselves and others.

Key signs and symptoms
- Euphoria
- Elevated mood
- Frustration, irritability, hostility
- Paranoia
- Delusions of grandeur
- Disinhibition
- Disturbed sleep pattern
- Pressure of speech
- Inability to concentrate, flight of ideas

Key history and assessment
- Previous history of hypomania, depression, or known bipolar disorder

Key observations and findings
- If possible a full set of vital signs helps ascertain physical impact of condition
- Patient may be uncooperative

Key investigations
- None required immediately
- Lithium levels can be checked if on lithium therapy

Key actions and treatment
- Mental health assessment required
- Neuroleptic drugs can help to calm the patient in the acute stage
- Lithium carbonate acts as a mood stabilizer in the longer term
- Security staff or police assistance may be required if patient is aggressive

⚙ Perceptual disorders (psychosis)

Perceptual disorders in mental health conditions can have a basis in reality whereby the form of an object is perceived in a manner that is different from its actual state. They may also take the form of hallucinations where objects occur entirely within the patient's imagination. Hallucinations may occur in any of the senses, with auditory and visual being most common. Hallucinations of smell, taste, or touch do occur in mental health conditions but may also indicate an underlying physical illness (such as temporal lobe epilepsy). All patients reporting or apparently experiencing perceptual disorders of any kind should have organic causes excluded.

! Panic disorder

Anxiety is a normal physical and psychological response to stress or perceived danger. Panic disorders are attacks of intense anxiety which can occur suddenly without warning and without an obvious stimulus. Fear of such attacks can lead to a low level of anxiety existing at all times. Anxiety can be part of another condition such as depression or alcohol abuse and may lead to the development of phobias. Panic attacks normally last <30min.

Physical manifestations include:
- Palpitations
- Chest pain or tightness
- Hyperventilation
- Choking sensation or feeling that their throat is closing
- Hot flushes, cold or hot sweats
- Dry mouth
- Nausea
- Dizziness
- Paraesthesia (resulting from hyperventilation)

Patients present as emergencies when they seek help during an attack or if a member of the public notices what is happening and summons help. Assessment should be focused on excluding underlying physical problems. Once this has been established no acute treatment is required during the attack other than reassurance. The patient should be referred to primary care for ongoing assessment and management once the acute attack has passed. Hyperventilation may be treated using a rebreather bag—a paper bag placed by the patient over their mouth in order to prevent excessive CO_2 loss which is responsible for dizziness and paraesthesia.

① Self-harm

Self-harm is not, of itself, indicative of a mental illness. The background to the event is normally complex and multifactorial. Anyone presenting having self-harmed will require a full assessment and evaluation.

📖 See Self-harm, p.361.

② Eating disorders

Anorexia nervosa and bulimia only become emergencies if the patient presents with associated physical problems. Usually patients can be referred for outpatient or primary care management as the conditions require ongoing support over a long period. Physical symptoms include weakness and cardiac arrhythmias resulting from hypokalaemia and seizures resulting from hyponatraemia. These problems should be identified and treated in the appropriate manner.

Neck pain

Differential diagnosis

☼ True emergencies
- Cervical spine injury
- Laryngeal injury
- Ludwig's angina
- Meningeal irritation
- Myocardial infarction

① Timely assessment
- Neck sprain (whiplash)
- Torticollis

Introduction

Most people will at some time suffer from neck pain. Minor strains occur as a result of overuse caused by physical activity. Stress and headache can also be associated with neck pain. Pain may also be the result of injury, degenerative conditions such as cervical spondylosis, or rheumatoid disease. Rarer causes include tumours and infections. Asking the patient to touch his/her chest with the chin is a simple screening test—inability to achieve this should alert one to the possibility of significant pathology. Weakness, altered sensation in the limbs or a change in bladder or bowel habit indicates possible spinal cord injury and requires urgent medical assessment.

☠ Cervical spine injury

Major or multiple trauma is the most common cause of cervical spine injury. The risk of an unstable spinal injury must be considered and managed in any patient presenting following high risk trauma (such as fall from a height, loss of consciousness following head injury, etc.). Neck injury and subsequent immobilization can be frightening for the patient. Clear explanations must be given at every stage of care. Staff should ensure they stand within the visual field of the patient to enable eye contact to be made while talking, without the patient having to move their head or neck. Aspects of cervical spine injury management are covered in the head injury guidance published by the National Institute for health and Clinical Excellence (NICE)[1].

Key signs and symptoms
- These depend on the level of the injury
- Neck or back pain
- Reduced range of movement in neck
- Alteration or loss of sensation
- Reduction or loss of motor function
- Inadequate or abnormal breathing

Key history and assessment
- Assessment should follow ABCDE principles of trauma management
- In suspected cervical spine injury the assessment should be as follows:
  - look
  - feel
  - XR
  - active movement
  - passive movement
- History of trauma
- Significant mechanism of injury:
  - fall from a height of >1m
  - collision at high speed
  - rollover motor accident
  - ejection from a motor vehicle
  - contact sport, such as rugby

- Multiple injuries
- Age ≥65 years
- Assess and document the extent of any altered sensation/motor function
- Locate any bony tenderness, whilst maintaining spinal alignment

Key observations and findings

- Respirations: may be inadequate or abnormal if a cervical cord injury is present
- SpO_2: may be reduced due to breathing difficulties
- Pulse: bradycardia (suggests cord injury) or tachycardia (suggests hypovolaemia)
- GCS should be documented. Reduced GCS may result from hypoxia, cardiovascular instability, or head injury
- Focal neurological deficit: weakness or reduced sensation
- BP: hypotension may occur secondary to cord injury or hypovolaemia

Key investigations

- XR appropriate to the location of the injury
- Lateral cervical spine XR
- Anterioposterior cervical spine XR
- Odontoid peg XR
- The base of skull, all seven cervical vertebrae, and T1 *must* be clearly seen on XR
- CT should be considered if also required for head injury, patients with multiple trauma, or when adequate XRs cannot be obtained

Key actions and treatment

- Requires immediate medical assessment
- Immobilize spine. This will require the use of a firm surface such as a spinal board outside of the hospital environment or a firm trolley in a clinical environment, head blocks, tape, and a semi-rigid cervical collar. This procedure should only be undertaken by trained staff
- Removal of spinal immobilization is a decision which should be made by an experienced clinician. The following criteria must be met:
  - GCS 15
  - adequate cervical spine imaging showing no fractures
  - no neurological deficit
- Manage airway as appropriate
- IV access and analgesia as appropriate
- IV fluid resuscitation if required
- Pressure area care will be required and limbs may need protecting
- Psychological support for the patient and their family

Further reading

1. National Institute for Clinical Excellence (2003). *Head Injury. Triage, assessment, investigation and early management of head injury in infants, children and adults.* London: NICE.

☠ Laryngeal injury

Injuries to the larynx are rare but can present with life-threatening airway problems. Both blunt and penetrating trauma can occur. The resulting swelling and deformity can cause partial or complete airway obstruction which is an airway emergency—*obtain immediate senior medical help if stridor is present*. Cervical spine injury must always be considered and managed until excluded.

Key signs and symptoms
- Obvious trauma
- Bruising and swelling
- Inspiratory noise—stridor
- Difficulty in swallowing saliva/drooling
- Hoarseness
- Neck pain
- SC emphysema
- Haemoptysis

Key history and assessment
- History of trauma and mechanism of injury
- Check adequacy of airway and breathing
- Check for neurological deficit

Key observations and findings
- Check adequacy of airway and breathing
- SpO_2: should be >94%
- Check for tachycardia: may result from hypoxia or hypovolaemia
- BP: should be normal unless significant blood loss has occurred
- Record GCS regularly

Key investigations
- CT neck
- Flexible fibreoptic laryngoscopy: requires specialist (ENT)

Key actions and treatments
- Check adequacy of airway and breathing
- Immediate senior medical assessment required if airway compromise is present
- Ensure airway is patent and secure
- Ensure adequate oxygenation
- High-flow O_2 via non-rebreathing mask, humidified if possible
- IV access for fluids, analgesia, and anaesthetic drugs
- Admit for ongoing management

☠ Ludwig's angina

A tense bilateral cellulitis of the submandibular, sublingual, and submental spaces which progresses rapidly. There is gross swelling of the neck and mouth. It is a potential airway emergency with a mortality rate of 75% if not treated rapidly.

📖 See Sore throat, p.391.

☠ Meningeal irritation

Inflammation of the membranes surrounding the brain and spinal cord which can be viral or bacterial in origin. The classical symptom of neck stiffness is often absent. The speed of progression of meningitis means it should not be overlooked in patients complaining of neck pain.

📖 See Headache, p.251.

☠ Myocardial infarction

The presence of pain radiating into the neck is well recognized as an indicator of myocardial ischaemia. Although patients usually have chest pain as well, on rare occasions they can present with isolated neck pain.

📖 See Chest pain, p.115.

⊙ **Neck sprain (whiplash)**

Hyperextension injuries as a result of rapid deceleration are common. Often referred to as whiplash, the term 'neck sprain' is preferred as it is more descriptive of the pathology.

Key signs and symptoms
- Neck pain which may radiate to shoulders and arms
- Neck stiffness and reduced range of movement
- Headache
- Backache

Key history and assessment
- History of rapid deceleration—usually minor road traffic collision
- Patient mobile since the incident
- No other significant injuries

Key observations and findings
- Restricted range of movement, particularly rotation
- Pain on palpation of neck muscles may be present
- No bony tenderness on palpation of the spinous processes
- No neurological signs or symptoms

Key investigations
- Usually none required
- Cervical spine XRs if:
  - severe mechanism of injury
  - pain immediately after the event
  - bony tenderness
  - other distracting injury

Key actions and treatment
- If any suspicion of bony or spinal cord injury apply semi-rigid collar and immobilize patient
- Oral non-steroidal anti-inflammatory analgesia
- Advise the patient to mobilize the neck normally; physiotherapy may be helpful
- Advise patient that symptoms may persist for several weeks
- *Soft neck collar should not be supplied as these delay healing*

⚠ **Torticollis**

Torticollis or wry neck is usually a minor self-limiting condition which occurs when the sternocleidomastoid muscle goes into spasm, twisting the neck and head over to one side. Rarely it can be a symptom of an underlying disease process and anyone with the following accompanying symptoms should be reviewed by a senior doctor urgently.

- Respiratory problems
- Neurological symptoms:
  - altered sensation in limbs
  - urinary incontinence
  - faecal incontinence
- Speech impairment or motor symptoms

Key signs and symptoms

- Head turned to one side
- Obvious spasm of a sternocleidomastoid muscle
- Pain
- Reduced range of movement

Key history and assessment

- Exclude recent trauma
- Exclude localized infection
- Exclude neck stiffness due to meningitis
- Consider drug induced dystonia

Key observations and findings

- Palpable and visible sternocleidomastoid muscle spasm

Key investigations

- If no history of trauma and no signs of underlying pathology then XR examination is not required

Key actions and treatment

- Oral medication:
  - anti-inflammatory medication
  - analgesia
- Locally applied heat
- Massage
- *Soft neck collar should not be supplied as these delay healing*

Overdose and poisoning

Differential diagnosis

☼ **True emergency**
- Cyanide

☼ **Urgent presentations**
- Alcohol
- Benzodiazepines
- Carbon monoxide poisoning
- Digoxin
- Opiates
- Paracetamol
- Salicylates
- Solvent inhalation
- Tricyclic antidepressants

Introduction

Overdose and poisoning can be accidental, an act of self-harm, or due to toxicity as a result of unwanted effects of prescribed medication. In accidental cases a full history of how the incident occurred should be obtained if possible. All patients presenting following self-harm should have a mental health assessment, provided that the drug/substance taken is not causing intoxication.

In all cases assessment should be made of:
- Substance or substances involved: confirmation should be obtained if possible from friends or relatives
- Quantity taken—if possible
- Time of ingestion
- Period over which ingestion occurred: single or staggered overdose
- Involvement of alcohol
- Physical symptoms
- Pre-existing medical/mental health problems
- Previous self-harm

In the UK information on a wide range of medicines, chemicals and other common substances can be obtained from the National Poisons Information Service via subscription to their online information service TOXBASE, or via telephone.

Emetics (such as ipecac) and gastric lavage are no longer recommended as treatment for overdose as there is no proven benefit and patients are therefore exposed to unnecessary discomfort and risk. Activated charcoal given in liquid form still plays a role in reducing the absorption of some substances if given within 1 hour of ingestion.

☠ Cyanide

Significant cyanide poisoning is rare and is most commonly seen in patients with smoke inhalation or following accidents in industrial processing. Cyanide (CN) is toxic by inhalation, ingestion, or contact. Inhalation of high concentrations of hydrogen cyanide can be fatal within a few minutes. Ingestion may lead to death within a few hours. Cyanide quickly detoxifies and any patients who are fully conscious and breathing normally after 5min following removal from exposure usually recovers without treatment.

Key signs and symptoms
- Dizziness
- Chest tightness
- Vomiting
- Headache
- Skin contact results in local irritation
- Anxiety
- Weakness
- Confusion, reduced level of consciousness
- Paralysis
- Seizures

Key history and assessment
- Exposure to processes using CN chemicals
- Evidence of smoke inhalation, ingestion or skin contact
- Length of time since exposure, length of exposure
- First aid given
- Assess for respiratory distress: especially pulmonary oedema
- Cardiac arrhythmias

Key observations and findings
- Pulse
- BP
- Respiratory rate
- GCS

Key investigations
- ABGs
- 12-lead ECG

Key actions and observations
- Avoid becoming contaminated and remove contaminated clothing
- Thoroughly wash patient's skin if there has been skin contamination
- Obtain senior medical assistance
- Ask patient to remove contact lenses if worn
- Give high-dose O_2 via a non-rebreathing mask, may require intubation and ventilating
- Establish IV access and IV fluids
- Continuous cardiac monitoring
- Regular recording of vital signs
- Admit for in-patient management, may need critical care
- Dicobalt edetate 300mg IV over 1min is the drug of choice for treatment in confirmed cases but must only be used in the presence of coma or respiratory depression as it is extremely toxic if no CN ions are present. Intubation equipment must be available

:⚙: **Alcohol**

Excessive alcohol intake places the patient at risk from injury, respiratory depression, aspiration of stomach contents and hypothermia.

Patients with a reduced level of consciousness require close monitoring and frequent assessment. A blood glucose measurement is mandatory as is a full set of vital signs, including GCS. Patients may require admission and consideration should be given to the need to treat for thiamine (vitamin B1) deficiency, which is common in alcohol abusers. Patients should only be discharged when they are sufficiently sober that they no longer present a risk to themselves.

📖 See Apparently drunk, p.37.

:⚙: **Benzodiazepines**

Used as tranquillizers and sedatives. When taken in overdose they are unlikely to cause any major long term effects. However if taken in conjunction with another depressant (e.g. alcohol) they can cause sedation and airway/respiratory problems. Patients who are asymptomatic at 4 hours post-ingestion are unlikely to experience any problems.

Key signs and symptoms
- Slurred speech
- Drowsiness/confusion
- Coma

Key history and assessment
- Amount taken
- Time taken and over what period
- Any alcohol taken
- Pre-existing mental health problems
- Pre-existing medical problems

Key observations
- Respiratory rate: reduced rate and inadequate breathing indicates severe poisoning
- BP: hypotension may occur
- Pulse
- SpO$_2$: may be reduced if respiratory depression is present

Key investigations
- ABGs: if GCS or SpO2 reduced
- Paracetamol: at 4 hours post-overdose and salicylate levels

Key action and treatment
- Protect the airway and maintain respirations if required
- Activated charcoal: if ingestion has occurred within 1 hour of presentation and the patient is able to maintain their own airway
- Obtain senior medical/anaesthetic assistance if respiratory problems are present or the patient is unresponsive

- *Do not give flumazenil*—as seizures can occur in mixed overdoses
- Refer to the in-patient medical team for ongoing management if necessary
- Provide supportive measures until the patient recovers
- Patients who become comatose normally spontaneously recover once the drug is metabolized as long as airway, breathing, and circulation are maintained
- Once physically stable refer to mental health team for assessment

☢: Carbon monoxide poisoning

CO is colourless, odourless and is produced during combustion where there is inadequate air supply (poorly maintained boilers, blocked flues, etc.). The gas diffuses easily into the blood where it binds with haemoglobin. CO has an affinity more than 200 × greater than O_2, forming carboxyhaemoglobin (COHb) which reduces O_2 carrying capacity with the blood. CO is known as a 'silent killer' as presenting symptoms are often vague. Always consider CO poisoning in patients who present with multiple vague symptoms.

Key signs and symptoms

- Signs of hypoxia without cyanosis
- Headache
- Dizziness
- N&V
- Syncope
- Weakness
- Reduced level of consciousness, confusion, coma
- Chest pain
- Arrhythmias
- Seizures

Key history and assessment

- Unexplained flu like symptoms or confusion
- Involved in fire in a confined space: especially if furniture or plastic burnt
- Inhalation of car exhaust fumes
- Faulty domestic gas appliance
- Use of chemical paint strippers in a confined space
- More than one person may be involved

Key observations and findings

- Pulse
- Respiratory rate
- BP
- GCS
- Pulse oximetry is unreliable as it can give a false reading due to the affinity to haemoglobin

Key investigations

- FBC, U&Es
- ABGs: metabolic acidosis in severe poisoning
- Check COHb level
- 12-lead ECG

Key actions and treatment

- Give high-flow O_2 via a non-rebreathing mask: high pO_2 will displace CO from haemoglobin more rapidly
- Regular vital sign observations including GCS
- Cardiac monitoring for arrhythmias

- IV access and fluids
- Control seizures if necessary
- Refer for admission and ongoing treatment
- Consider hyperbaric O_2 therapy if neurological or cardiac problems occur or the patient is pregnant: senior medical review is required

☼ Digoxin

Self-harm with digoxin is unusual, but it has a low therapeutic index and therefore toxicity with therapeutic doses can occur.

Key signs and symptoms
- Anorexia
- Nausea
- Vomiting
- Visual problems
- Confusion
- Collapse

Key history and assessment
- Based on symptoms
- Other medications, increased risk with some drug interactions
- Assess for cardiac failure or arrhythmias
- Other medical conditions

Key observations
- Pulse: irregular, bradycardia
- BP: hypotension
- Respiratory rate
- Monitor SpO$_2$
- Temperature
- GCS

Key investigations
- U&Es: hypokalaemia exacerbates toxicity
- Digoxin levels
- 12-lead ECG

Key actions and treatment
- Depends on level of toxicity
- Nausea only, occasional ventricular ectopics:
  - stop digoxin for 2–3 days
  - if potassium low, then prescription of oral potassium 20–40mmol daily
  - will require reassessment within 3 days
- Any other symptoms:
  - IV access
  - continuous cardiac monitoring
  - manage any arrhythmias as appropriate
  - experienced medical review required—may require IV potassium, IV magnesium or digoxin-specific Fab (DSF(ab)) therapy

:O: Opiates

Overdose with opiates may occur via oral or IV routes.

Key signs and symptoms
- Altered level of consciousness, confusion, aggression, coma
- Nausea/vomiting
- Pin-point pupils

Key history and assessment
- Substances taken and when
- Any other substance taken
- Pre-existing medical conditions

Key observations and findings
- Respiratory rate: reduced rate and adequacy
- SpO_2
- Pulse: bradycardia is common
- BP: hypotension is common
- Temperature: may be hypothermic

Key investigations
- None usually required

Key actions and treatments
- Maintain airway and assist breathing if required
- IV access—if possible
- Naloxone 0.4mg IV/IM, can be repeated at 2-min intervals if required
- Observe until stable
- Caution with long-acting opiates (such as methadone) as the effect of naloxone will wear off within an hour and toxicity can reoccur
- Refer to substance abuse team if appropriate

:⚙: Paracetamol

Paracetamol is the most common medication taken in overdose in the UK. The most serious complication of paracetamol poisoning is hepatic failure which may occur within 2–3 days of a severe overdose. In some patients (e.g. those with low body mass and pre-existing liver disease) toxicity may occur with relatively small quantities of ingested paracetamol.

Key signs and symptoms
- Often asymptomatic in the first 24 hours
- Early signs:
  - N&V
  - loss of appetite
  - abdominal pain
- Later signs:
  - hypoglycaemia
  - haemorrhage
  - altered consciousness level, confusion, coma
  - cardiac arrhythmias

Key history and assessment
- Type of preparation taken: plain paracetamol or combination product
- Amount taken and when
- Any other drugs/alcohol taken
- Pre-existing medical problems
- Previous overdoses

Key observations and findings
- Baseline vital signs

Key investigations
- Paracetamol levels should be taken at 4 hours post-ingestion—earlier testing is unreliable. However this is only useful for a single overdose—'staggered' overdoses produce unreliable paracetamol levels
- FBC, U&Es, LFTs
- INR: if overdose >24 hours previously

Key actions and treatment
- Oral activated charcoal can be given within 1 hour of ingestion in order to reduce absorption
- Need for treatment depends on paracetamol levels and time since ingestion
- If indicated, IV N-acetylcysteine (NAC) can be given according to a treatment nomogram
- Admit for ongoing treatment
- If patient presents later than 24 hours admit for further assessment and management
- If no medical treatment is indicated refer for mental health assessment

☼ Salicylates

Overdose of aspirin can result in a complex medical picture depending upon the quantity ingested.

Key signs and symptoms
- Vomiting
- Sweating
- Epigastric pain
- Tinnitus
- Deafness
- Altered level of consciousness, confusion, coma
- Seizures

Key history and assessment
- Preparation taken and quantity
- Time taken
- Alcohol or other drugs taken
- Pre-existing medical problems
- Any previous overdoses

Key observations and findings
- Pulse: tachycardia
- Temperature: pyrexial/hyperpyrexia
- BP: hypo or hypertension
- GCS: for level of consciousness

Key investigations
- U&Es
- Paracetamol and salicylate levels: repeat salicylate levels every 2 hours until they start to fall
- ABGs
- Blood glucose

Key actions and treatment
- If <1 hour since ingestion give activated charcoal to reduce absorption
- Refer to in-patient medical team for ongoing assessment and management

☼ Solvent inhalation

Solvent inhalation may occur accidentally through the use of chemicals in a confined space without adequate ventilation or the absence of correct personal protective equipment. Alternatively inhalation may be a form of substance misuse. Collapse may occur as a result of intoxication, hypotension or cardiac arrhythmias. Patients may also develop hypoxia due to aspiration of stomach contents or the solvent itself.

Key signs and symptoms
- Altered level of consciousness
- Hallucinations
- Vomiting
- Headache
- Dizziness
- Smell of solvent of breath/clothing
- Rash or spots around the nose and mouth may indicate chronic abuse

Key history and assessment
- Substance involved, length of exposure
- Deliberate or accidental

Key observations and findings
- Pulse
- Respiratory rate: may be depressed or laboured
- SpO_2
- GCS

Key investigations
- May require ABGs if respiratory inadequacy is present
- 12-lead ECG

Key actions and treatments
- Maintain airway and breathing
- High-flow O_2 therapy via a non-rebreathing mask
- Continuous cardiac monitoring for arrhythmias
- If patient's condition fails to improve refer to in-patient medical team
- Refer to substance misuse team if available or mental health team

:☼: Tricyclic antidepressants

Tricyclic antidepressants (TCA) are used in the treatment of depression, anxiety disorders, and some forms of chronic pain. Toxicity results from anticholinergic effects—tachycardia, dilated pupils, urine retention, drowsiness and seizures. Death can occur from respiratory depression, cardiac arrest, or prolonged seizures.

Key signs and symptoms
- Dilated pupils
- Dry mouth
- Urinary retention
- Altered levels of consciousness, drowsiness, confusion, coma
- Seizures

Key history and assessment
- Quantity taken, time taken, and over what period of time?
- Any alcohol or other drugs taken?
- Pre-existing mental health problems
- Pre-existing medical problems
- Any previous overdoses?

Key observations and findings
- Pulse: tachycardia
- Respiratory rate
- SpO_2
- BP
- GCS: must be regularly assessed
- Pupillary assessment: often dilated

Key investigations
- FBC, U&Es, ABGs
- Tricyclic levels
- 12-lead ECG for signs of cardiac toxicity

Key actions and treatments
- Urgent medical review required
- Protect and maintain airway if level consciousness reduced: intubation may be required to secure the airway
- Within 1 hour of ingestion activated charcoal may be used to reduce absorption provided the patient is not drowsy—beware of the risk of aspiration should the patient become unconscious
- ECG monitoring is essential
- IV access required
- Sodium bicarbonate may be required under the direction of senior medical officer
- Admission to ITU for ongoing monitoring and assessment is often required
- If patient is clinically well refer to mental health team for assessment

Palpitations

Differential diagnosis

⚙ True emergencies
- Broad complex tachycardia

⚙ Urgent presentations
- Narrow complex tachycardia

Introduction

The sensation of being aware of the heart beat is normal during periods of exertion or anxiety. However palpitations may occur at rest and these require investigation ± treatment.

The patient may describe irregular, fast, abnormally forceful, slow or 'missed' beats. Causes of palpitations include:
• Anxiety
• Excessive use of stimulants such as caffeine, nicotine, and alcohol
• Withdrawal from the use of stimulants
• Unwanted effects of drug therapy—e.g. doxazosin
• Hyperthyroidism
• Cardiac arrhythmias: primary or secondary to ischaemia etc.

The main priority in management is to identify and manage any clinically significant arrhythmias. These can be divided into broad complex (usually ventricular tachycardia) and narrow complex arrhythmias.

A 12-lead ECG can be helpful, but may miss an intermittent arrhythmia. Continuous monitoring using 3-lead electrodes is more reliable.

Associated symptoms which give cause for concern are:
• Shortness of breath
• Chest tightness
• Chest pain
• Dizziness
• Syncope

If no obvious cause is found for the palpitations from the history and examination, blood tests may be taken for FBC, U&Es (especially potassium levels) and TFTs.

If the patient is well and no cardiac problems are identified then discharge and primary care follow-up may be considered. If in doubt, discuss with a physician. Patient should be advised to reduce exposure to known triggers such as caffeine, alcohol etc.

☠ Broad complex tachycardias

Ventricular tachycardia

The most serious cause of palpitations is VT which appears as a regular broad complex tachycardia (usually >130/min). VT is a clinical emergency as it has the potential to progress to cardiac arrest (pulseless VT or VF). Short runs of VT may be asymptomatic; longer lasting episodes cause symptoms related to a reduced cardiac output (low BP, angina, dyspnoea, confusion, etc.).

Causes include:
- Ischemic heart disease
- Structural abnormalities such as cardiomyopathy
- Complication of anti-arrhythmic drug therapy
- Electrolyte imbalance
- Hypoxia

VT can be sub-divided according to the clinical condition of the patient:
- Stable: clinically well, normal BP, no pain or dyspnoea
- Unstable: alert but unwell, may have reduced BP, pain, or dyspnoea
- Cardiac arrest: pulseless VT

Stable ventricular tachycardia

The patient is well and has no chest pain, no dyspnoea, and BP is >100mmHg systolic, their condition can be considered as stable. However, urgent treatment is still required in order to prevent clinical deterioration.

Key actions and treatment
- Urgent medical referral required
- Ensure airway and breathing are adequate
- High-flow O_2 via a non-rebreathing mask
- Continuous cardiac monitoring via defibrillator
- IV access
- Frequent observation of pulse, BP, respiratory rate, and SpO_2

Unstable ventricular tachycardia

If a pulse is present the patient's clinical condition should be assessed urgently. If any of the following are present the patient's condition should be considered as unstable.

Key signs and symptoms
- Chest pain
- Tachycardia >150bpm
- Systolic BP <90mmHg
- Altered level of consciousness
- Dyspnoea

Key history and assessment
- In the presence of adverse signs or symptoms treatment should commence prior to obtaining a history

Key observations and findings
- Pulse rate
- BP
- SpO_2
- GCS

Key investigations
- Continuous cardiac monitoring via a defibrillator
- 12-lead ECG if patients condition allows
- U&E, cardiac enzymes, blood glucose, ABGs

Key actions and treatment
- Immediate assessment by senior medical staff required
- Anaesthetic support may be required
- Ensure adequate airway and breathing
- High-flow O_2 via a non-rebreathing mask
- IV access
- Synchronized DC cardioversion under conscious sedation is required
- Full explanations should be given to the patient
- Patient requires admission to a HDU—e.g. CCU

Pulseless ventricular tachycardia

The patient presents in cardiac arrest.

Key signs and symptoms
- Collapse
- Unresponsiveness
- No pulse

Key history and assessment
- Assess for signs of life

Key observations and findings
- Assess cardiac rhythm via a defibrillator

Key investigations
- None at this point

Key actions and treatment
- Commence advanced life support according to Resuscitation Council (UK) guidelines[1]

Further reading

1. Resuscitation Council (UK) (2005). *Resuscitation Guidelines 2005*. London: Resuscitation Council (UK).

:✪: **Narrow complex tachycardia**

A narrow QRS complex is one which lasts <0.12sec (3 small squares on standard ECG paper). These arrhythmias may be classified as regular or irregular as below:

Regular arrhythmias
- Common conditions
  - supraventricular tachycardia (SVT)
  - atrial flutter
- Vagal manoeuvres should be attempted first:
  - only attempt one manoeuvre; if it fails, others are unlikely to be successful. Examples include:
    —valsalva manoeuvre (patient closes mouth, holds nostrils closed and attempts to breath out forcefully)
    —carotid sinus massage (maximum of 15sec, attempt on one side only)
- If unsuccessful:
  - adenosine 6mg bolus
  - repeat (with 12mg) up to three times if sinus rhythm is not restored
  - if unsuccessful experienced medical review required

Irregular arrhythmias
- Atrial fibrillation (AF). This is the most common cardiac arrhythmia with incidence increasing with age
- Disorganized atrial activity occurs with irregular ventricular contractions resulting. This produces the classically 'irregularly irregular' pulse of AF
- If the condition last >48 hours there is significant risk of:
  - embolic stroke
  - medical advice required.
- If <48 hours since onset then IV amiodarone 300mg followed by 900mg over 24 hours with the aim of restoring sinus rhythm
- If >48 hours since onset then anticoagulation will be required (if not already on warfarin) prior to attempting to control rate/rhythm

Further reading

National Institute for Clinical Excellence (2006). *Clinical guideline 36. The management of atrial fibrillation.* London: NICE.

Pregnancy

Differential diagnosis

True emergencies

- Eclampsia
- Ectopic pregnancy
- Emergency childbirth
- Placental abruption
- Trauma

Urgent presentations

- Miscarriage
- Placenta previa
- Pre-eclampisa
- Premature rupture of membranes

Introduction

Normal pregnancy is considered to last around 40 weeks and is divided into 3 trimesters. When caring for a pregnant patient, in addition to the history of the presenting complaint, the previous obstetric history should also be obtained. This should include recording gravidity (total number of pregnancies) and parity (number of completed pregnancies). Gestation of previous births should be recorded along with the type of delivery, birth weight, and any significant antenatal or post-partum events. The expected date of delivery should be noted along with results of ultrasound scans and laboratory tests. Many women will have patient-held notes which may contain useful information. It is important to remember at all times that you are dealing with two patients.

Vaginal bleeding is a common presentation during pregnancy. It is important to confirm the bleeding is pregnancy related and not the result of trauma, infection, or other cause (Table 32.1).

Vaginal examinations should only be performed by staff who are trained in the procedure and are able to make definitive clinical decisions.

The emotional and psychological impact of problems in pregnancy should be considered and sensitive support provided.

Table 32.1 Causes of vaginal bleeding in pregnancy

First trimester	Second trimester	Third trimester
Ectopic pregnancy	Miscarriage	Placental abruption
Miscarriage	Trophoblastic disease	Placenta previa
Trophoblastic disease	Placental abruption	Pregnancy show
	Placenta previa	

:☠: Eclampsia

Eclampsia is a condition of unknown aetiology, normally occurring in patients who have suffered from pre-eclampsia. It is defined as the onset of seizures after the 20th week of pregnancy associated with hypertension and protein-uria (however it can occur without proteinuria and with a minimal increase in BP). The maternal mortality rate is believed to be somewhere between 10–35% and the fetal mortality rate between 15–30%.

Key signs and symptoms
- Fitting
- Reduced level of consciousness
- Evidence of end-organ failure:
  - hypertension
  - proteinuria
  - upper limb or facial oedema
  - headache
  - visual disturbances
  - abdominal pain
  - acute renal failure

Key history and assessment
- 20th week and later gestation
- Recent delivery: 20–25% of cases occur post-partum; although 98% of these occur in the first 24 hours, it can occur up to 3 weeks after delivery
- First-time mother
- <20 or >35 years
- History of pre-eclampsia/eclampsia
- Pre-existing medical condition:
  - diabetes
  - hypertension
  - renal disease

Key observations and findings
- Pulse
- BP
- Respiratory rate
- Cardiac monitoring
- GCS

Key investigations
- Blood glucose
- Urinalysis

Key actions and treatment
- Immediate medical help is required
- Maintain airway
- High-flow O_2 via a non-rebreathing mask
- Anticonvulsant therapy: magnesium sulphate 4g IV as a loading dose, then 1–4g per hour as an infusion
- Emergency referral to obstetric team

☠ Ectopic pregnancy

A pregnancy occurring anywhere outside the uterus is termed ectopic—it is also known as an extrauterine pregnancy. The most common location is within a fallopian tube that has become blocked or inflamed, although the fetus can also become attached to the cervix or an ovary. In the vast majority of cases the woman will miscarry. Problems arise when the growth of the fetus causes bleeding from associated structures. The haemorrhage may be life threatening if undiagnosed or if there is a delay in treatment. Ectopic pregnancy normally occurs between the 6–12th week of pregnancy. Patients may not be aware of the pregnancy—it is therefore important to perform a pregnancy test in all women of childbearing age who present with abdominal pain.

Key signs and symptoms

- Symptoms may be mild at first, becoming worse as the tube swells and then ruptures
- Missed period
- Abnormal vaginal bleeding
- Normal signs of pregnancy may be present
- Lower abdominal, suprapubic pain—may localize to shoulder tip
- Pale, clammy, sweating
- Collapse

Key history and assessment

- Many women have no identifiable risk factors
- Risk increases with age
- Previous pelvic inflammatory disease
- Previous ectopic pregnancy
- Tubal surgery
- Previous terminations: risk higher if >2 terminations
- Undergoing in-vitro fertilization
- Intrauterine device (IUD) in situ

Key observations and findings

- Respiratory rate: tachypnoea if significant haemorrhage has occurred
- O_2 saturation should be monitored
- Pulse: tachycardia due to internal haemorrhage or pain
- BP: hypotensive suggests haemorrhage
- Continuous cardiac monitoring for potential life-threatening arrhythmias
- Temperature: usually normal

Key investigations

- Urine pregnancy (beta-human chorionic gonadotropin (βhCG)) test: a negative test *does not* exclude an ectopic pregnancy
- Serum βhCG test: always positive
- Bloods:
  - FBC: check Hb
  - U&Es: baseline renal function
  - group and save/cross match as appropriate
- Ultrasound: to differentiate between viable pregnancy, miscarriage, or ectopic

Key actions and treatment

- Immediate medical assessment
- High-dose O_2 via a non-rebreathing mask
- Wide-bore IV access in both arms
- Pain relief with IV morphine titrated to pain and vital signs
- If haemodynamically unstable, fluid resuscitation and stabilization
- May require urgent transfer for surgery
- Psychological support for patient and family. Patients are often scared and anxious for both themselves and for the pregnancy
- Explain to patient and family there is no possibility of saving the 'baby'/pregnancy

☠ Emergency childbirth

Healthcare professionals may be faced with a woman in the late stages of labour for a number of reasons, including multiparous women whose labour progresses quicker than they anticipated or those who have concealed pregnancy.

Key signs and symptoms
- Contractions
- 'Show': small vaginal bleed
- Rupture of amniotic membranes: waters breaking

Key history and assessment
- Gestation of pregnancy
- Parity
- History of the progress of previous deliveries

Key observations and findings
- Frequency and duration of contractions
- Note extent of cervical dilatation
- Pulse
- Respiratory rate
- BP

Key actions and treatment
- Call for help:
  - wherever there is the possibility of emergency childbirth occurring, local arrangements should be in place
  - in a hospital setting this may involve pre-agreed arrangements to call a combination of midwife, obstetrician, anaesthetist, paediatrician, as required
  - in the community setting this may involve transporting a midwife or GP to the patient
  - emergency transportation of the patient via ambulance to a maternity unit may be required
- Allow the women to adopt a position in which she is comfortable
- Provide analgesia nitrous oxide 50% and O_2 50% (Entonox®) if possible
- Attention should be paid to ensure the umbilical cord is not around the baby's neck, if it is a finger should be slipped between the cord and the neck and an attempt should be made to manoeuvre it over the head
- Support the head without placing any pressure on it
- The baby should be dried and wrapped in a warm blanket or towel immediately
- Record the Apgar score at 1 and 5min (Table 32.2)
- Record time of birth

The Apgar score
The Apgar score was developed by Dr Apgar in 1953 (Table 32.2):
- **A**: Appearance
- **P**: Pulse
- **G**: Grimace
- **A**: Activity
- **R**: Respiratory effort

An Apgar score between 7–10 requires no action. Between 4–7 needs intervention, normally suctioning and supplemental O_2; <4 requires active resuscitation.

Table 32.2 The Apgar score

Factor	Score		
	0	1	2
Heart rate	Absent	<100	>100
Respirations	Absent	Slow, irregular	Strong cry
Muscle tone	Limp	Some flexion of limbs	Good flexion
Colour	Blue	Blue hands and feet, pink body	Pink
Reflex	Absent	Some motion	Good motion

☠ Placental abruption

Abruption is defined as separation of the placenta due to haemorrhage after the 20th week of gestation. Maternal and fetal death may occur due to haemorrhage or coagulopathy.

Key signs and symptoms
- Bleeding after 20 weeks: may range from mild loss to major haemorrhage
- Abdominal pain
- Back pain
- Uterine pain: often severe
- Abnormal contractions
- Premature labour

Key history and assessment
- Older mother: >35 years
- Trauma
- Tobacco smoking
- Post amniocentesis

Key observations and findings
- Pulse
- BP
- Respiratory rate
- O_2 saturation
- Amount of blood loss
- Severity of pain

Key investigations
- FBC
- U&Es
- Blood glucose
- Clotting screen
- Group and save/cross-match as required
- Rhesus status
- Kleihauer test
- Ultrasound

Key actions and treatment
- High-flow O_2 via a non-rebreathing mask
- Commence fluid resuscitation if required
- Monitor vital signs
- Fetal monitoring will be required
- Urgent referral to obstetrician

:☣: Trauma

It is estimated that up to 10% of pregnant women experience some form of trauma with the majority occurring in the third trimester. Trauma is usually minor in nature. Road traffic collisions account for 60% of the major trauma cases, with the majority of other serious injuries occurring as a result of falls or assault, including domestic violence. In penetrating trauma the fetus is injured in up to 70% of incidents.

The pregnant patient presents difficult clinical problems as two lives need to be considered. However the focus must be on the mother as 80% of traumatic fetal deaths result from maternal hypovolaemia. This may occur as a result of pelvic fractures, splenic and hepatic injuries. Traumatic haemorrhage can also result from placental abruption where rapid deceleration tears the placenta from the wall of the uterus.

The anatomical and physiological changes which occur in pregnancy can make assessment difficult. The uterus moves out of the pelvis in week 12. It is highly resistant to trauma, rarely rupturing, and provides some level of protection to the other displaced abdominal organs.

In the third trimester the uterus can cause compression of the inferior vena cava resulting in circulatory collapse. This can be alleviated by wedging the patient in a left lateral position. If this cannot be achieved due to the possibility of a spinal injury then the uterus should be manually displaced.

Key signs and symptoms
- History of recent trauma
- Vaginal bleeding
- Premature rupture of membranes

Key history and assessment
- The mechanism of injury needs to be fully understood so the risks to the patient and the fetus can be assessed
- Major trauma patients requires assessment by senior emergency care staff and an obstetrician
- LMP
- Estimated date of confinement (EDC)
- Assess for fetal movement if at an appropriate stage of the pregnancy
- Assess for uterine contractions
- Ascertain if a seatbelt was being worn if the incident was a road traffic collision
- Assessment of the abdomen for pain and tenderness is unreliable in the later stages due to peritoneal stretching
- Consider the risk of domestic violence in vague or inconsistent histories
- Assess location and extent of any bruising

Key observations and findings
- During pregnancy the pulse may be slightly raised and BP reduced when compared with the patient's normal readings
- However, in the setting of trauma, hypotension or tachycardia should be assumed to be secondary to haemorrhage until proven otherwise

Key investigations
- The use of investigations will depend on the extent of trauma, the clinical needs of the mother, and the relative risk to the fetus
- Ultrasound is the most useful investigation in the majority of cases to examine for haemorrhage and fetal heart movement
- Unnecessary XRs should be avoided. If possible the fetus should be protected with lead shielding
- FBC
- U&E
- Blood group and save/cross match according to clinical condition
- Kleihauer–Betke test detects fetal-to-maternal hemorrhage. A positive test may indicate life-threatening hemorrhage in the fetal circulation
- Urinalysis

Key actions and treatment
- In major trauma experienced medical help is required
- The first actions should be aimed at stabilizing the mother
- Assessment of the fetus should be undertaken as part of the secondary survey and urgent referral made to an obstetrician
- High-flow O_2 is required due to the high risk of fetal hypoxia
- Large bore IV cannula required
- IV fluids as needed to maintain adequate circulation
- Give anti-D immunoglobulin if abdominal trauma is present and the mother is Rh– to prevent the formation of antibodies if the baby is Rh+
- Patients <20 weeks' gestation with minor trauma do not require specific intervention or monitoring, but the anxiety experienced by the patient should not be underestimated and may be relieved by referral to a midwife for assessment of the pregnancy

☼ Miscarriage

Miscarriage is the loss of a pregnancy before 24 weeks' gestation. The most common time for miscarrying is between 6–10th week of gestation. Miscarriage is more common in women >30 years of age. Estimates of the frequency of pregnancies ending in miscarriage vary from 1 in 4 to 1 in 8. The main requirements are to ensure haemodynamic stability, pain relief and psychological care.

Classification of miscarriage

- Threatened:
  - up to 14 weeks
  - intermittent bleeding
  - cervical os closed
  - mild cramping pain
  - no fetal tissue passed
- Inevitable:
  - heavy bleeding
  - cervical os open >5mm
  - persistent cramping pain, moderate-to-severe
  - no fetal tissue passed
- Incomplete:
  - heavy bleeding with clots
  - cervical os open
  - severe abdominal pain
  - fetal tissue passed or visible
- Complete:
  - light bleeding
  - cervical os closed
  - mild or no pain
  - fetal tissue passed
- Missed:
  - no bleeding or brown vaginal discharge
  - cervical os closed
  - mild or no pain
  - no fetal tissue passed
  - risk of infection
- Septic:
  - uncommon
  - varied blood loss
  - offensive discharge
  - cervical os open
  - may have passed fetal tissue
  - moderate to severe pain
  - pyrexia

Key signs and symptoms

- Type and amount of bleeding:
  - number of pads used
  - fresh or dark blood
  - clots passed

- fetal tissue passed
- stage of bleeding: light then heavy or heavy becoming lighter
- Nature and severity of pain:
  - location
  - severity
  - often described as cramps
  - progression of pain: getting worse or lessening

Key history and assessment

- Age of patient
- Obstetric history:
  - significant events in previous pregnancy
  - progression of this pregnancy
  - previous miscarriage

Key observations and findings

- Ensure patient is haemodynamically stable:
  - pulse
  - respiratory rate
  - BP
- Temperature

Key investigations

- Urine sample to confirm pregnancy
- Exclude urinary infection
- Ultrasound to check for:
  - viable pregnancy
  - retained products of conception
- Consider the need for a FBC and group and save if heavy blood loss

Key actions and treatment

- Depends on type of miscarriage and status of patient
- If required obtain medical assistance
- O_2 15L/min via a non-rebreathing mask
- IV fluids if heavy bleeding
- Pain relief
- Check Rh status: if Rh− will need prophylactic anti-D gammaglobulin if over 12 weeks or undergoing surgery
- Refer to gynaecology team

Psychological care

The emotional and psychological aspects of miscarriage should be considered. Sensitive use of language and the provision of clear information may help, as will a compassionate approach and acknowledgement of the feelings the woman is experiencing. Many patients report undergoing a grieving process following a miscarriage, as well as a period of depression, loneliness, and isolation. Self-blame, anger, and jealousy of other pregnant women are also common reactions which can be very difficult to deal with. Many areas have local support groups which can be helpful in supporting women and their partner in coming to terms with their loss.

☼ Placenta previa

Failure of the placenta to move away from the opening to the cervix during the development of a pregnancy occurs in about 0.2–0.5% of pregnancies, with the risk doubling in multiple pregnancy—twins or triplets—and also increasing with each subsequent pregnancy. In women who have had routine antenatal care it is usually detected on ultrasound. Presentation for emergency care may be early in the pregnancy as a result of anxiety related to spotting, or towards the end of the pregnancy during to severe bleeding or premature labour.

Key signs and symptoms
- Spotting of blood during the first two trimesters
- Moderate to heavy bleeding in the third trimester, after 28 weeks
- Bleeding is normally painless
- May experience contractions during the bleeding

Key history and assessment
- Previous Caesarean section is the most significant risk factor
- Previous history of placenta previa
- Aged >35 years
- Smoking
- Previous dilation and curettage (D&C) or other uterine surgery

Key observations and findings
- Amount of blood loss
- Pulse, BP, respiratory rate: for signs of hypovolaemia

Key investigations
- Ultrasound if patient presents early in her pregnancy will confirm the position of the placenta

Key actions and treatment
- Depends on the stage of the pregnancy, the amount of bleeding, and if bleeding is still occurring
- Early treatment is aimed at ensuring that any blood loss is managed appropriately and the pregnancy is maintained
- Emergency treatment in the third trimester is aimed at ensuring the patient survives any blood loss and the birth is as controlled as possible. The patient will probably require a Caesarean section
- Emergency referral to an obstetrician will be required
- Assess for signs of labour

☼ Pre-eclampsia

Defined as pregnancy-induced hypertension, pre-eclampsia is the most common serious complication in pregnancy and must not be confused with mild hypertension which may occur without significant risk. For pre-eclampsia to be diagnosed the hypertension needs to be combined with either proteinuria or facial/upper limb oedema. Estimates of its frequency vary between 1:7 and 1:14 pregnancies and estimates of those developing the most severe form vary between 1:50 and 1:100.

Key signs and symptoms
- Oedema: facial/upper limbs
- Headache
- Visual disturbances
- Right-sided upper abdominal pain
- Vomiting

Key history and assessment
- Gestation: more common after 20 weeks
- First-time mother or first pregnancy with this partner
- Age:
  - <20 or >35 years
- Multiple pregnancies: expecting twins or more
- Pre-existing medical condition:
  - diabetes
  - hypertension
  - renal disease
- Family history
- Obesity

Key observations and findings
- Hypertension:
  - systolic 30mmHg above patient's norm
  - diastolic 15mmHg above patient's norm

Key investigations
- Protein in urine (proteinuria)

Key actions and treatment
- IV magnesium sulphate
- Refer to obstetrics for monitoring
- 📖 See Eclampsia, p.335, for further information

✸ **Premature rupture of membranes**

Premature rupture of membranes (PROM) occurs in approximately 10% of pregnancies with 2% occurring before 37 weeks. It is these early cases which may be considered an emergency if there is significant leakage of amniotic fluid or any indications of infection. The reason for the rupture is often unknown but infection, STDs, smoking, and previous pre-term births are all thought to increase risk. Once the membranes have ruptured, delivery usually occurs within the week. Other risks include infection of the placenta, placental abruption, umbilical cord compression, and post-partum infection.

Key signs and symptoms
- Sudden passing of watery fluid from the vagina
- Persistent leakage of amniotic fluid
- Abdominal pain
- Vaginal bleeding

Key history and assessment
- History should include previous pregnancies and health during this current pregnancy
- Vaginal examination should *not* be undertaken due to the risk of introducing infection

Key observations and findings
- Pulse: should be normal but may be raised due to stress or potential infection
- BP and respiratory rate: should be normal
- Check for pyrexia due to infection, often low grade
- Fetal tachycardia: seen on Doppler ultrasound

Key investigations
- FBC
- Mid-stream urine
- Blood cultures
- Ultrasound for gestational age
- Cervical swab for bacterial infection

Key actions and treatment
- Refer for an obstetric opinion
- May require admission
- Psychological support of the mother and partner

Further reading

Arulkumaran S (2006). *Emergencies in Obstetrics and Gynaecology*. Oxford: Oxford University Press.

62 Premature rupture of membranes

PV bleeding

Differential diagnosis

:✪: **Urgent presentations**
- Bleeding in pregnancy

① **Timely assessment**
- Traumatic bleeding

⑦ **Non-urgent presentations**
- Abnormal menstruation
- Reproductive age bleeding
- Peri-menopausal bleeding
- Post-menopausal bleeding

Introduction

Patients with PV bleeding rarely present as emergencies unless:
- It occurs as a result of trauma
- It is severe enough for the patient to be systemically unwell
- It is so abnormal the patient feels an emergency assessment is required
- The patient wishes to be assessed by someone other than their normal healthcare practitioner

On emergency presentation the healthcare practitioner should establish:
- Has the patient experienced abnormal PV bleeding previously?
- Estimation of blood lost: number of tampons/towels/pads used
- Type of bleeding: menstrual, fresh bleeding, presence of clots
- Timing of bleeding: irregular, relationship to menstrual cycle, post-coital
- LMP date
- Contraceptive history: note particularly any recent changes
- Previous gynaecological and obstetric history
- Indications of hypovolaemia: tachycardia, hypotension, tachypnoea
- Presence of other symptoms: pelvic pain, weight loss, persistent abdominal distention
- History of trauma/assault
- A pregnancy test should be undertaken on all patients to exclude ectopic pregnancy, or other pregnancy-related bleeding
- Consideration should be given to doing a FBC to exclude anaemia before discharge

If it can be established that the patient is haemodynamically stable, the bleeding not the result of trauma, and pain management is addressed, she may be referred to her primary care physician as long-term management and investigation is likely to be required.

If not as a result of trauma, PV bleeding can be categorized into one of five different groups which are based on reproductive status:
- Bleeding during pregnancy
- Abnormal menstruation
- Reproductive-age bleeding
- Peri-menopausal bleeding
- Post-menopausal bleeding

☼ Bleeding in pregnancy

Bleeding in pregnancy can be an extremely worrying event. In some cases it may give no further cause for concern; however, it may be indicative of a number of problems including miscarriage, ectopic pregnancy, placental abruption, or placenta praevia.

📖 See Pregnancy, p.333.

① Traumatic bleeding

The most common cause of vaginal trauma is consensual intercourse. Trauma may occur as a result of insufficient lubrication or personal sexual preferences. Insertion of FBs into the vagina may also cause trauma. It is important to exclude abuse. The patient should be given privacy and time in which to discuss these issues should she wish. Straddle injuries, where the patient falls aside an object such as a bicycle, can result in lacerations and trauma to the vagina has also been reported following the use of water slides, where the hydrostatic pressure can cause lacerations. All but the most minor of vaginal lacerations require an expert review.

⑦ Abnormal menstruation

Heavy menstrual bleeding (menorrhagia) is a problem which requires long-term management and the development of an understanding of the needs and expectations of the patient. Patients should be referred to their primary care physician for assessment, investigation, and management. Patients may present to the emergency setting with symptoms of anaemia.

⑦ Reproductive age bleeding

Most commonly indicative of a benign condition such as PID or endometrial polyps. Bleeding can occasionally be a sign of malignant disease. Use of the oral contraceptive pill (OCP) may also cause irregular breakthrough bleeding when it is first used or if it is changed. Unless patients are clinically unwell they should be referred to their primary care practitioner.

⊘ Peri-menopausal bleeding

The menopause usually occurs between the ages of 47–53. Bleeding in the peri-menopausal years either side of actual menopause can quite often be irregular due to anovulatory cycles in which ovulation does not occur as changes in hormone levels interfere with the process. Unless patients are clinically unwell they should be referred to their primary care practitioner.

⊘ Post-menopausal bleeding

Bleeding after the onset of the menopause needs to be investigated in primary care. Hormone replacement therapy (HRT), infection, benign polyps, or atrophy of the endometrium may all cause bleeding. However, a number of malignant causes may also be responsible.

Rashes

Differential diagnosis

☼ **Emergency presentations**

- Septicaemia

⏲ **Timely assessment**

- Allergies
- Cellulitis

⦿ **Non-urgent presentations**

- Contact dermatitis
- Drug reactions
- Fungal infections
- Heat rash
- Scabies
- Sexually transmitted disease
- Shingles

Introduction

A number of conditions have an accompanying rash with the vast majority being minor. However, the presence of a rash may be indicative of a serious medical condition. Due to public awareness of conditions such as meningococcal septicaemia patients presenting with rashes are common in emergency care settings. There are a number of key aspects within the history/assessment which are common to all patients with a rash.

Key history and assessment

- Is there any itching, discomfort, or pain?
- Any blistering, ulcers, dry flaky skin, or discharges?
- On which part of the body did the rash first appear?
- Where has the rash spread to?
- When did the rash first appear?
- Is the rash getting better or worse?
- Where was the patient when the rash first occurred?
- What was the patient doing when the rash first appeared?
- What is the patient's occupation?
- Have they had a similar condition before?
- Is anyone else affected?
- Any treatment tried?
- Type and features of rash—e.g. bullae, pustules, petechiae, purpura?

☠ Septicaemia

Septicaemia—the presence of actively dividing bacteria within the blood—may be associated with a rash. Septicaemia is a medical emergency which requires emergency antibiotic treatment. The patient will be systemically unwell and requires immediate medical attention.

The presence of a classic purpuric, non-blanching rash in an unwell patient is highly suggestive of meningococcal septicaemia. Purpura is caused by blood leaking into the tissues and appears at first like small pinpricks which develop rapidly into larger bruises. However it is important to note that early in the presentation the rash may blanch and be maculopapular in nature.

In addition it should be noted that meningococcal septicaemia may occur in the absence of meningococcal meningitis. Readers are encouraged to familiarize themselves with current UK meningitis guidelines.

📖 See Headache, p.251.

Key signs and symptoms
- Sudden onset of fever
- Rash; petechiae; pinpoint, red flat spots which don't blanch when pressed; purpura, similar to petechiae but covering a larger area and more purple in colour
- Irritable and agitated
- Altered level of consciousness
- Cold and clammy

Key history and assessment
- Recent history of infection.
- Contaminated/infected wound

Key observations
- Continuous cardiac monitoring
- Pulse
- Respiratory rate, tachypnoea or dyspnoea
- BP: hypotension is an important sign
- Temperature

Key investigations
- FBC, U&Es, LFT, clotting factors
- ABGs
- Blood and urine for bacterial C&S

Key actions and treatment
- Immediate medical intervention: will require ITU if hypotensive or respiratory distress present
- High-flow O_2 therapy 15L via non-rebreathing mask
- IV access: large-bore cannulae × 2 if possible
- IV fluids
- IV antibiotics according to guidelines

⚠ Allergies

The presence of raised, erythematous, itchy lesions, usually referred to as urticaria' or 'hives' are a feature of many allergic reactions. They are a response to histamine release and in most cases cause nothing more than discomfort. They may, however, become widespread and indicate the onset of an anaphylactic reaction which requires immediate medical intervention.

📖 See Allergy, p.31.

! Cellulitis

Bacterial infection of the dermis and SC tissues normally caused by streptococci or staphylococci which penetrate the skin barrier. Most patients respond well to oral antibiotic treatment in the community but those at increased risk (e.g. diabetics) or who present late may require hospitalization.

Key signs and symptoms
- Localised redness
- Affected area warm to touch
- Swelling to the affected area
- Pain on movement or palpation
- Swollen lymph nodes

Key history and assessment
- Assess for probable source
  - history of recent trauma
  - concurrent skin condition—eczema, psoriasis
- Assess for risk factors: pre-existing medical condition—diabetes, steroids, lymphoma etc.
- Assess for complications:
  - systemic involvement
  - abscess formation
  - orbital cellulitis
  - signs of osteomyelitis

Key observations
- Vital signs as a baseline and to ensure no systemic involvement:
  - temperature—may be pyrexial, responsive to antipyretics
  - pulse
  - respiratory rate
  - BP

Key investigations
- None initially

Key actions and treatments
- Oral antibiotics according to local guidelines
- Analgesia for pain and pyrexia: paracetamol or NSAIDs
- Advise rest
- Elevation of affected limb will help to reduce swelling
- If signs of systemic involvement present then refer for medical assessment

⑦ Contact dermatitis

Contact dermatitis can either be allergic or irritant—caused by contact with an irritant material. In the allergic condition the patient may have a history of allergies including to the current trigger. Common substances include nickel (jewellry), latex, cosmetics, and perfumes. In irritant contact dermatitis the rash is red and itchy and may appear like a superficial burn in more serious exposures. Avoidance of the trigger is the best management although this may not always be possible. Topical corticosteroids may help.

⑦ Drug reactions

Many prescribed medications can produce an erythematous reaction. Antibiotics are amongst the most common. The patient should be referred back to the clinician who prescribed the medication for further advice.

⑦ Fungal infections

Fungal infection can be transmitted from animals as well as people. Common conditions include athlete's foot and ringworm. They cause a dry, itchy, scaling rash which commonly occurs in the groin, on the trunk, or on the feet. Treatment is usually with antifungal preparations and is applied topically.

⑦ Heat rash

Heat rash or prickly heat is caused by sweat glands becoming blocked by dead skin cells or bacteria in hot weather when profuse sweating occurs. The rash, small red papules, will usually last for several days and commonly occurs on the hands, feet, under arms, and across the chest. The patient experiences an itching or prickly sensation and blistering may be present. Heat rash normally clears without treatment within 2–3 days but may last longer if the weather is hot or humid. Oral antihistamines may help; however, ointments and lotions may make the condition worse by further blocking sweat glands.

⑦ Scabies

Scabies is caused by infestation by the scabies mite (*Sarcoptes scabiei*). The condition is spread by close contact, shared clothing or bedding. The female mite tunnels under the skin laying eggs. This results in visible burrows 2–10mm long especially in web spaces, wrists, elbows, armpits, and under breasts. The symptoms are due to an allergic reaction and can take several weeks to develop. The allergic rash, which is blotchy in appearance, can spread diffusely, most often to the inner thighs, abdomen, and ankles, although the infestation is localized. Skin can become secondarily infected by bacteria. Treatment is with permethrin cream 5% or malathion liquid. All close contacts should be treated and the patient warned that the itch may continue after treatment for up to 3 weeks.

⑦ Sexually transmitted disease

A number of STDs can present with a rash. Genital ulcers and sores may result from infection with herpes virus, papilloma virus, or syphilis. Once STD is suspected treatment, investigation and ongoing management is more appropriately undertaken in a GUM clinic.

⑦ Shingles

Following primary infection with chicken pox, the varicella-zoster virus remains dormant within the dorsal ganglion of a sensory nerve. At a later stage, often when a patient is unwell for other reasons, the virus may reactivate and cause a vesicular rash in the distribution of that nerve. The rash appears similar to that of chicken pox other than its highly localized distribution. The pain experienced by the patient may be severe and can occur 2–3 days before the rash. Antiviral medication (aciclovir 800mg, 5 times a day for 7 days) may be prescribed to limit the severity of the condition and analgesia will be required.

Self-harm

Differential diagnosis

:☺: **True emergencies**
- Altered conscious level
- Major haemorrhage

:✿: **Urgent presentations**
- Ingestion of objects
- Self-poisoning

① **Timely assessment**
- Incisions

Introduction

Self-harm is very common, particularly in the young. The reasons are often complex and multi-factorial, with the individual not always fully understanding his/her own behaviour. Underlying feelings of rage, aggression, low esteem, helplessness, emptiness, and grief have all been described. Some patients report a sensation of relief or release following self-harm.

History of physical, sexual, and psychological abuse is very common amongst this group of patients. In addition, substance misuse or mental health problems are also often present.

There are three main groupings of self-harm which result in patients presenting for emergency care:
- Traumatic acts of high lethality:
  - jumping from heights
  - hanging
  - car crashing
  - self-inflicted burns
  - jumping in front of moving vehicles
  - gunshot
- Poisoning and overdose:
  - medications—prescription or OTC
  - illicit drugs
  - CO
  - household and industrial chemicals
- Self-mutilation:
  - superficial minor burns
  - self-inflicted cuts
  - ingestion/insertion of objects

A further group of self-harming behaviours are more subtle. These include:
- Eating disorders: anorexia/bulimia
- Addictive behaviours: alcohol/substance misuse
- Risk-taking lifestyle

The first priority should always be the assessment and treatment of the injury or illness itself. If the condition is assessed as non-life- or limb- threatening then psychosocial assessment/intervention can take place.

All people who have self-harmed require detailed assessment of:
- The amount of distress displayed
- Evidence of mental illness
- Suicidal intent
- Trigger for current episode
- Social circumstances and needs
- Feelings of hopelessness or powerlessness

All these factors should be taken into account when deciding ongoing management. Where possible referral to other services should be made with the patient's knowledge and agreement.

Older patients should be seen by clinicians experienced in managing mental health problems in the elderly and particular attention should be paid to:
• Evidence of depressive illness
• Pre-existing medical problems and their impact on the patient
• Cognitive function

If the patient does not wish to stay for further assessment their capacity to make this decision should be assessed and clearly documented. Their primary care physician and Mental Health Services should be informed in order to enable suitable follow-up to be offered. If the patient is assessed as lacking capacity an in-depth mental health assessment will be required. If they are unwilling to wait for this, consideration should be given to preventing them from leaving by using the appropriate legislation—staff need to be familiar with the appropriate sections of the Mental Health Act.

Admission should be considered for patients who meet the following criteria:
• Severe psychological distress
• Patient under the influence of drugs or alcohol
• Lack of a safe home environment

Suicidal intent

There is a strong relationship between previous self-harm and suicide. As part of the assessment of self-harm, consideration should be given to suicidal intent. Patients should be asked about their intention to further self-harm or to commit suicide. Asking these questions does not increase the risk of further action.

The presence of any of the following indicators in a patient who has self-harmed significantly increases the risk of a successful suicide attempt in the future:
• History of mental illness
• Saving tablets to overdose
• Organizing finances/making a will
• Previous acts of self-harm
• Failure to seeking help following previous self-harm
• Recent bereavement
• Overwhelming financial problems
• Feelings of worthlessness/hopelessness regarding the future
• Workplace stressors
• Pre-existing physical illness
• Substance/alcohol abuse
• Family history of suicide

A number of tools are available to help assess those patients at risk of attempting suicide, including the Beck Hopelessness Scale,[1] the SAD PERSON scale,[2] and the Australian Mental Health Triage Scale[3].

The SAD PERSONS Scale is a 10-point tool with one point being allocated for each positive answer. The higher the number scored, the higher the risk of suicide attempt:
• **S**ex, males at higher risk
• **A**ge, young adults or very old 75+

- **D**epression
- **P**revious attempt
- **E**thanol abuse
- **R**ational thinking loss, psychosis
- **S**ocial support lacking
- **O**rganized plan
- **N**o spouse
- **S**ickness, chronic illness

The Australian Mental Health Triage Scale[3] provides three groupings of risk:
- Immediate risk:
  - attempted hanging
  - self-inflicted gun shot wound
  - CO poisoning
  - serious laceration requiring suture
  - requiring medical treatment beyond activated charcoal or routine neurological observation
  - requiring admission to a CCU
  - major psychiatric illness/psychosis
  - evidence of serious suicide intent
- Serious risk:
  - evidence of psychiatric illness such as depression, schizophrenia, personality disorder
  - history of psychiatric illness and treatment
  - alcohol or drug abuse
  - previous suicide attempt
  - access to a firearm
  - chronic physical illness
  - evidence of continuing suicidal ideation or intent
- Lesser risk:
  - first episode of deliberate self-harm
  - no evidence of major psychiatric disorder
  - no evidence of continuing suicidal ideation or intent
  - no history of drug or alcohol abuse
  - evidence that the crisis has resolved

Criteria should be established with local Mental Health Services regarding the actions to be taken depending on the results of the assessment.

Further reading

1. Beck AT (1988). *Beck Hopelessness Scale*. San Antonio: The Psychological Corporation.
2. Patterson WM, Dohn HH, Bird J, *et al.* (1983). Evaluation of suicidal patients: The SAD PERSON Scale. *Psychosomatics*, **24**(4), 343–9.
3. Australasian College for Emergency Medicine and The Royal Australian and New Zealand College of Psychiatrists (2000). *Guidelines for the Management of Deliberate Self Harm in Young People*. Carlton/Melbourne: Australasian College for Emergency Medicine, Royal Australian and New Zealand College of Psychiatrists.
4. National Institute for Clinical Excellence (2004). *Self-harm. The short-term physical and psychological management and secondary prevention of self-harm in primary and secondary care*. London: NICE.

☠️ Altered conscious level

Any patient who presents with a decreased level of consciousness following self-harm requires immediate medical intervention.

📖 See Collapse, p.131.

☠️ Major haemorrhage

Any act of self-harm which results in major haemorrhage requires immediate medical intervention to prevent the development of hypovolaemic shock and a critical life-threatening condition.

📖 See Major trauma, p.293.

☠️ Ingestion of objects

A variety of objects may be ingested. The primary objective is to ensure that the object has not been aspirated and that the patient's airway is clear. Once the object has reached the stomach it is likely to pass through the GI tract uneventfully.

📖 See Foreign bodies, p.233.

☠️ Self-poisoning

Drug overdose is the most common method of self-harm. However, self-poisoning may involve other materials including household/industrial chemicals and CO. These should all be considered as medical emergencies and managed appropriately prior to a psychiatric assessment.

📖 See Overdose and poisoning, p.313.

⚠ Incisions

Self-inflicted incisions are a relatively common presentation for emergency care. These wounds are rarely life or limb threatening. Often they follow a pattern as indicated:

- Multiple wounds in easily accessible sites—e.g. forearm
- Wounds of varying depth indicating hesitation
- Signs of previous self-inflicted incisions

The wounds should be managed appropriately prior to psychiatric assessment

📖 See Wounds, p.427.

Shortness of breath

Differential diagnosis

☺ True emergencies
- Airway obstruction
- Anaphylaxis
- Asthma
- Haemothorax
- Myocardial infarction
- Pneumothorax
- Pulmonary embolism

☼ Urgent presentations
- Acute bronchitis
- Blunt trauma
- Chronic obstructive pulmonary disease
- Heart failure
- Hyperventilation
- Pleurisy
- Pneumonia

ⓘ Timely assessment
- Anaemia
- Malignancy

Introduction

Shortness of breath (dyspnoea) is a common emergency presentation and is a symptom of many different medical conditions, both acute and chronic.

Most cases of acute shortness of breath are due to lung and breathing disorders, cardiovascular disease, or chest trauma. It is a condition which some patients may experience many times due to recurrent acute exacerbations of chronic diseases. This may result in a familiarity with the condition which can lead to a delay in seeking medical assistance and complacency on the part of the healthcare professional in the provision of treatment and care.

Each episode of dyspnoea should be assessed with reference to any pre-existing respiratory condition, and consideration should be given to previous treatment and progression of earlier acute events.

☠ Airway obstruction

Ensuring a patient's airway is clear is the first priority whenever a clinical assessment is undertaken. Without adequate oxygenation and ventilation the patient will suffer irreversible hypoxic brain injury within 4min.

Causes of airway obstruction
- Trauma:
  - blunt
  - penetrating
  - inhalation injuries
  - chemical burns
- FB
- Anaphylaxis: angioedema
- Infection:
  - epiglottitis
  - laryngitis

Key signs and symptoms
- Obvious respiratory distress
- Recurrent coughing in an effort to clear obstruction
- Visible blood or vomit obstructing the airway
- Stridor
- Paradoxical chest/abdominal movements indicates severe obstruction
- Cyanosis
- Agitation
- Altered conscious level
- Dysphonia/inability to speak
- Trauma to the face or neck
- Swelling to the neck

Key history and assessment
- *It is essential to clear the airway if possible before attempting to obtain a detailed history*
- Is there a history of trauma and, if so, what mechanism was involved?

- History of allergies?
- Any recent infection, sore throat, or dental pain?
- Relevant medical history
- Auscultate chest

Key observations and findings
- Respiratory rate, rhythm, effort, ability to speak
- Pulse: usually tachycardic
- O_2 saturation: urgent intervention needed if SpO_2 <94%
- BP
- Cardiac monitoring: high risk of arrhythmias / cardiac arrest
- Temperature

Key investigations
- *Treatment must take priority over any investigations*
- Once airway is secure and breathing stabilized:
  - ABGs
  - FBC
  - U&Es
  - Glucose
  - CXR

Key actions and treatment
- Inspect patient's mouth for obvious foreign material—*do not perform a 'blind sweep'*

If FB present:
- Lean patient forward and encourage coughing
- If visible, remove FB
- If patient cannot clear obstruction by coughing:
  - stand behind the patient to one side, support the chest with one hand, give 5 sharp blows between the shoulder blades with the heel of your other hand
  - check mouth again

If unsuccessful:
- Summon immediate medical help: anaesthetic or ENT if available
- Stand directly behind the patient
- With the patient leaning forward:
  - place your fist between the umbilicus and the sternum with your thumb resting on the patients abdomen (see Fig. 36.1)
  - holding your fist with your other hand pull sharply upwards and inwards 5 times
  - check the mouth again
  - repeat if necessary until help arrives

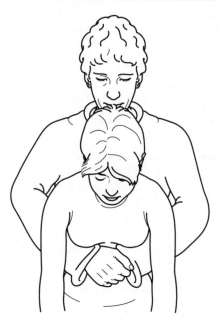

Fig. 36.1 Abdominal thrust

☠ Anaphylaxis

Anaphylaxis is an abnormal reaction to an allergen. At its most extreme anaphylaxis can cause swelling of the soft tissues of the face, mouth, and upper airways, including the larynx, which can result in airway obstruction. Bronchospasm and mucus secretion also occur, resulting in narrowing of the lower airways, further exacerbating the patient's dyspnoea.

📖 See Allergy, p.31.

☠ Asthma

Asthma is a chronic inflammatory disease of the airways. Exacerbations occur as a result of exposure to an allergen which causes bronchospasm and mucus secretion. This results in coughing, wheeze, and dyspnoea. Asthma is a common condition affecting approximately 5% of adults. Throughout the world death rates from asthma continue to rise, with around 1500 fatalities occurring in the UK each year.

📖 See Asthma, p.53.

☠ Haemothorax

Accumulation of blood within the pleural cavity may occur following trauma. The signs, symptoms, and the treatment required will depend upon the severity of the haemorrhage and subsequent compression of the lung and chest cavity contents.

📖 See Torso injury, p.405.

☠ Myocardial infarction

Up to 10% of patients suffering acute MI will present with dyspnoea as their main symptom. All patients complaining of dyspnoea should have a 12-lead ECG recorded and the diagnosis of MI considered.

📖 See Chest pain, p.115.

☠ Pneumothorax

Pneumothorax can be caused by trauma or may occur spontaneously—particularly where there is underlying chronic chest disease. The fluid seal between the visceral and parietal layers of the pleural cavity is broken and air rushes into the space created resulting in a partial or complete collapse of the lung.

A tension pneumothorax is a life-threatening condition. The damaged area of the lung creates a one-way 'flap' valve which allows air into the pleural cavity each time the patient breathes in, but prevents air from exiting when the patient breathes out (Fig. 36.2). This gradually 'inflates' the pleural cavity causing compression of chest contents. Cardio-respiratory function is severely compromised and, if untreated, cardiac and respiratory arrest will follow.

Key signs and symptoms

Spontaneous pneumothorax
- Sudden onset of unilateral pleuritic chest pain
- Dyspnoea
- Cough
- Tachycardia, tachypnoea
- Reduced air entry on affected side

Tension pneumothorax
- Tachypnoea
- Absent breath sounds on affected side
- Tracheal deviation away from the affected side
- Tachycardia: >130/min
- Hypotension
- Distended neck veins
- Collapse/cardiorespiratory arrest

Key history and assessment
- Spontaneous: young, tall, thin males are typically affected
- Secondary:
  - elderly patients
  - COPD
  - asthma
- Infections:
  - pneumonia
  - lung abscess
- Trauma: blunt or penetrating
- Iatrogenic:
  - after pleural biopsy or aspiration
  - subclavian vein cannulation
  - mechanical ventilation

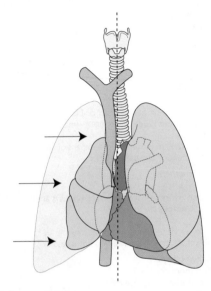

Fig. 36.2 Tension pneumothorax

Key observations and findings
- Pleuritic chest pain
- Dyspnoea
- Cough
- Hyper-resonance to percussion
- Diminished breath sounds on the affected side
- Tracheal deviation: tension pneumothorax
- Hypoxia
- Tachycardia

Key investigations
- Tension pneumothorax is a clinical diagnosis and requires intervention prior to XR
- Erect expiratory CXR—if tension pneumothorax is not suspected
- Pulse oximetry

Key actions and treatment

- Referral to medical team: immediate or urgent depending on clinical condition
- The British Thoracic Society has published guidelines for the management of spontaneous pneumothorax[1] (Figs. 36.3 and 36.4)

Small pneumothorax

- Small rim of air at the apex
- Analgesia:
  - simple oral analgesia, paracetamol or NSAIDs are often sufficient
  - do not use nitrous oxide (Entonox®)—may increase size of pneumothorax
- Will require review to ensure that re-expansion has occurred. This may be on an in-patient or out-patient basis

Moderate pneumothorax

- Analgesia:
  - simple oral analgesia, paracetamol or NSAIDs are often sufficient
  - do not use nitrous oxide (Entonox®)
- O_2
- Aspiration of air via a cannula and three-way tap
- May require chest drain if aspiration is unsuccessful

Complete pneumothorax

- 'Empty' hemithorax on CXR
- Cardiac monitoring with pulse oximetry
- Regular recording of vital signs
- High-flow O_2 through a non-rebreathing mask
- Analgesia:
  - simple oral analgesia, paracetamol or NSAIDs are often sufficient
  - do not use nitrous oxide (Entonox®)
- Chest drain

Tension pneumothorax

- Requires immediate treatment
- High-flow O_2 via a non-rebreathing mask
- Decompress tension pneumothorax, needle thoracocentesis:
  - insert a 14–16G IV cannula perpendicular to the chest
  - 2nd intercostal space, mid-clavicular line
- Chest drain required as soon as possible
- CXR following chest drain insertion

Open pneumothorax

Open pneumothorax is commonly caused by penetrating chest trauma, although it may also occur with high impact blunt chest trauma. The patient presents with acute respiratory distress due to the lung collapsing and with a visible chest wound. The patient may be haemodynamically unstable and will require a primary survey and active resuscitation.

📖 See Major trauma, p.293.

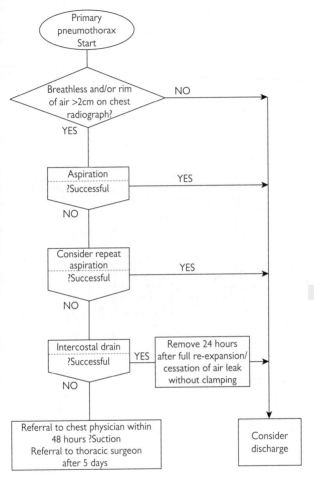

Fig. 36.3 Guidelines for treatment of primary pneumothorax. Reproduced with permission from The British Thoracic Society.

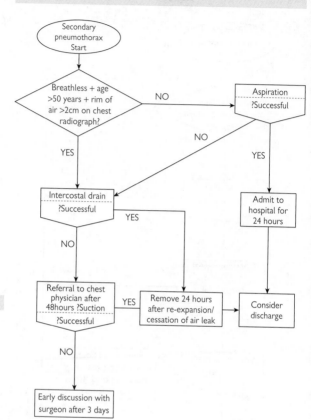

Fig. 36.4 Guidelines for treatment of secondary pneumothorax. Reproduced with permission from The British Thoracic Society.

Further reading

1. Henry M, Arnold T, Harvey J, *et al.* (2003). BTS guidelines for the management of spontaneous pneumothorax. *Thorax*, **58** (suppl II), ii39–ii52.

:☼: Pulmonary embolism (PE)

A PE causes the total or partial obstruction of a pulmonary artery—usually caused by a blood clot, although they can also rarely be caused by fat or air. Gas exchange within the lung is compromised and a ventilation perfusion mismatch occurs. The risks for PE are similar to those for DVT including surgery, immobility, neoplasia, and pregnancy.

PE can be classified into massive or non-massive according to the degree of vascular obstruction caused—massive PE will result in a significant drop in BP and patient collapse.

Key signs and symptoms

- Sudden onset of breathlessness
- Chest pain: sharp or pleuritic—may be absent in massive PE
- Cough
- Cyanosis
- Haemoptysis
- Collapse
- Anxiety or restlessness
- Reduced level of consciousness

Key history and assessment

- Previous history of PE or DVT
- Heart disease especially:
  - heart failure
  - AF
  - prosthetic valves
- Pregnancy or recent childbirth
- Obesity
- Malignant disease
- Period of immobilization:
  - surgery, especially hip or abdominal within 14 days
  - bed rest
  - long distance journeys, especially planes
  - lower-limb plaster cast

Key observations and findings

- Dyspnoea
- Tachypnoea
- Pulse oximetry
- Tachycardia
- Hypotension
- Prolonged capillary refill

Key investigations

- ABGs
- CXR: to exclude other causes of dyspnoea
- ECG: may show heart strain in massive PE
- CT pulmonary angiogram (CT-PA) is the investigation of choice
- Ventilation/perfusion scan (VQ)

Key actions and treatment
- Immediate medical support required
- Resuscitate if necessary
- Sit patient upright if possible
- High concentration O_2 through a non-rebreathing mask
- IV access
- Regular vital signs observation
- Cardiac monitoring
- Give analgesia as required
- Treat any cardiac arrhythmias which occur
- IV fluids
- Anticoagulate with heparin
- Thrombolysis may be indicated if massive pulmonary embolus is diagnosed

⚙ Acute bronchitis

Acute bronchitis is normally a self-limiting illness which can be treated at home with rest, simple analgesics, and antipyrexial drugs.

Key signs and symptoms
- Cough
- Sore throat
- Pyrexia: mild
- Wheeze
- Sputum production: may be initially clear, becoming purulent with bacterial superinfection
- Dyspnoea: with more severe infection

Key history and assessment
- URTI
- General malaise
- Higher risk for serious infection if:
  - pre-existing chest disease
  - immunosuppressed
  - cardiac conditions
  - smoker
  - reduced mobility

Key observations and findings
- Vital signs usually normal
- Wheeze may be present
- Pyrexia: mild

Key investigations
- Normally none required as diagnosis can be made on clinical grounds

Key actions and treatment
- Analgesics and antipyrexial drugs: normally paracetamol
- Advise rest
- Antibiotics not normally required
- If patient is systemically unwell consider:
  - additional O_2 support
  - IV antibiotics
  - reconsider diagnosis
  - refer for admission

⚙ Blunt trauma

Although blunt chest trauma is a relatively common presentation (either as an isolated injury or in conjunction with multiple trauma) anyone who experiences associated shortness of breath requires careful assessment to determine the cause. Management is focused upon identifying serious underlying injuries such as haemorrhage, cardiac, or pulmonary injuries.

📖 See Major trauma, p.293.

☼ Chronic obstructive pulmonary disease

COPD is the accepted term for diseases characterized by slowly progressive airflow obstruction which is not completely reversible by medical intervention. Smoking is the major causative factor although occupational exposures to other hazards can also play a role in its development.

Emergency care may be sought for acute exacerbations of COPD where the patient's condition deteriorates acutely from the normal. In a significant proportion of acute exacerbations no causative factor can be found. Current evidence suggests that the majority of these acute events are triggered by viral infections. Less frequent causes include bacterial infections and atmospheric pollutants.

Key signs and symptoms
- Increased productive cough
- Progressive dyspnoea/respiratory distress
- Wheeze unrelieved by inhalers
- Change in sputum colour
- Cyanosis
- Confusion suggests severe exacerbation
- Chest pain and haemoptysis are uncommon and consideration should be given to other causes for the shortness of breath

Key history and assessment
- History of COPD
- Smoking history—this is best expressed in pack years:
  - number of cigarettes smoked per day
  - divided by 20
  - multiplied by the number of years smoked
- Normal level of mobility

Key observations and findings
- The degree of breathlessness related to activities is a key observation in COPD. This can be measured using the MRC dyspnoea scale:[1]
  - 1: not troubled by breathlessness except on strenuous exercise
  - 2: short of breath when hurrying or walking up a slight hill
  - 3: walks slower than contemporaries on the level because of breathlessness, or has to stop for breath when walking at own pace
  - 4: stops for breath after about 100m or after a few min on the level
  - 5: too breathless to leave the house, or breathless when dressing or undressing
- Pulse may be high in presence of bacterial infection and/or hypoxia
- Respiratory rate usually elevated
- Temperature may be raised in the presence of bacterial infection
- SaO_2 is often reduced
- Level of consciousness may be reduced if the patient has a severe exacerbation of their condition
- Wheeze

Key investigations

- Patients with mild exacerbations may be managed without investigations
- More serious exacerbations may require:
  - CXR
  - ABGs: repeated to monitor response to treatment
  - FBC, U&Es, sputum culture
  - 12-lead ECG
  - Peak flow rate: check what is normal for the patient

Key actions and treatment

- NICE guidelines indicate criteria for hospital admission (Table 36.1)[2]
- Nurse patient sitting upright
- Monitor closely for respiratory depression
- SpO_2 should be maintained between 90–93%
- O_2 therapy if patient is hypoxic and systemically unwell; commence with high flow O_2 and monitor ABG. If in doubt, obtain medical advice
- Monitor cardiac rhythm
- Antibiotics may be required if consolidation is seen on CXR
- Bronchodilators may be given via a nebulizer
- Oral corticosteroids
- If patient fails to improve within 30min then senior medical review is required

Table 36.1 Criteria for hospital admission

Factor	Home	Hospital
Able to cope at home	Yes	No
Breathlessness	Mild	Severe
General condition	Good	Poor/deteriorating
Level of activity	Good	Poor/confined to bed
Cyanosis	No	Yes
Worsening peripheral oedema	No	Yes
Level of consciousness	Normal	Impaired
Receiving long-term O_2 therapy	No	Yes
Social circumstances	Good	Lives alone/not coping
Acute confusion	No	Yes
Rapid rate of onset	No	Yes
Significant comorbidity—particularly cardiac disease and insulin-dependent diabetes	No	Yes
SaO_2 <90%	No	Yes
Changes on CXR	No	Present
Arterial pH level	≥7.35	<7.35
Arterial PaO_2	≥7kPa	<7kPa

Further reading

1. Medical Research Council Dyspnoea Scale. Adapted from: Fletcher CM Elmes PC, Fairburn MB (1959). The significance of respiratory symptoms and the diagnosis of chronic bronchitis in a working population. *British Medical Journal*, **2**, 257–66.

2. National Institute for Clinical Excellence (2004). Clinical Guideline 12. Chronic obstructive pulmonary disease: management of chronic obstructive pulmonary disease in adults in primary and secondary care. London: NICE.

☼ Heart failure

Heart failure may be acute or chronic. Left ventricular failure (LVF) is the commonest emergency presentation. The left ventricle loses the ability to pump effectively, pressure increases in the pulmonary veins, causing fluid to be 'squeezed' into the alveolar spaces—pulmonary oedema. This inhibits O_2 absorption causing dyspnoea and hypoxia. In 90% of cases LVF occurs as a result of coronary artery disease or hypertension.

Key signs and symptoms
- Dyspnoea
- Orthopnoea—breathlessness worsened on lying flat
- Pink frothy sputum
- Sweating/clammy
- Pallor
- Anxiety
- Chest tightness or pain
- Cyanosis

Key history and assessment
- Time of onset of symptoms
- Waking at night with breathlessness
- Previous medical history
- Reduced mobility due to dyspnoea
- Breathlessness worse when lying flat
- Persistent cough

Key observations and findings
- Dyspnoea and tachypnoea
- Tachycardic
- Reduced O_2 saturation: serious problem if <94%
- BP: usually hypertensive in acute LVF
- Continuous cardiac monitoring required due to the risk of cardiac arrhythmias
- Basal crackles

Key investigations
- Treatment may need to be commenced before any investigations are undertaken
- CXR helps to confirm diagnosis
- 12-lead ECG may reveal acute ischaemic changes
- ABG
- U&E, glucose, cardiac enzymes

Key actions and treatment
- Position patient upright
- High-flow O_2 via non-rebreathing mask
- Urgent medical intervention required
- IV access needed

- Drugs used for LVF work by causing vasodilatation. This reduces the pressure in the blood vessels, and will encourage the return of oedematous fluid to the intravascular space. Common examples are:
  - nitrates
  - diuretics
- If no improvement CPAP may be required under medical direction

☼ Hyperventilation

Hyperventilation is a behavioural response to anxiety which results in inappropriate 'over-breathing'. The term 'hyperventilation' is *not* appropriate for a physiological response to conditions such as DKA, hypovolaemia, etc. The diagnosis should not be made until physiological causes have been excluded.

Hypoventilation results in a reduction of the $PaCO_2$ which is the cause of the signs/symptoms of the condition.

Key signs and symptoms
- Rapid, shallow respirations
- Cramp and spasm in hands and feet
- Feeling of lightheadedness
- Palpitations
- Chest tightness
- Dry mouth and difficulty swallowing

Key history and assessment
- History of anxiety
- Previous presentations with hyperventilation
- No other medical reason for tachypnoea

Key observations and findings
- Respiration rate, tachypnoea
- Pulse rate, tachycardia
- SpO_2: normal

Key investigations
- None required

Key actions and treatment
- Explain the nature of the condition to the patient
- Use of a 'rebreathing' bag will alleviate symptoms by causing the patient to rebreathe exhaled gases and thereby increasing his/her $PaCO_2$. The simplest method utilizes a paper bag which the patient places over the mouth and nose into which they breathe
- Explore the reasons for the anxiety attack and refer the patient for stress management if appropriate

⚙ **Pleurisy**

Pleurisy occurs when the membranes between the lungs and the chest wall (pleura) become inflamed. Patients present with pain which is exacerbated by inspiration. The condition may be caused by infection (such as pneumonia), pulmonary embolism or some connective tissue diseases (e.g. rheumatoid disease).

Key signs and symptoms
- Pain on inspiration
- Difficulty in taking a deep breath or coughing
- Pyrexia may occur where infection is the cause

Key history and assessment
- Symptoms suggestive of chest infection
- History of connective tissue disease
- Symptoms suggestive of DVT/PE

Key observations and findings
- Temperature
- Pulse
- BP
- Respiration rate
- Monitor O_2 saturation

Key investigations
- Diagnosis is based on clinical history and examination
- CXR may help confirm an underlying pneumonia
- DVT or PE may need to be excluded

Key actions and treatment
- Anti-inflammatory drugs (such as ibuprofen or diclofenac) may be used to ease pain and inflammation
- Antibiotics may be required if bacterial infection is confirmed

☼ Pneumonia

Pneumonia is normally caused by a bacterial infection of the lung. Some patients (particularly young adults) can be managed in the community whereas others will require admission to hospital. A number of factors are associated with higher mortality including the presence of concurrent medical conditions, immunosuppression, and old age. Pneumonia may present with confusion or collapse in the elderly and must be considered in the differential diagnosis of these patients.

Key signs and symptoms
- Cough: dry or productive
- Purulent sputum or haemoptysis
- Dyspnoea
- Pyrexia
- Dehydration especially in the elderly
- General malaise
- Confusion

Key history and assessment
- Recent URTI
- Dullness to percussion
- Crackles on auscultation over the affected area
- History of smoking and/or alcohol abuse
- Chronic systemic illness
- Pre-existing lung disease

Key observations and findings
- Respiratory rate usually elevated
- Heart rate: tachycardia is common
- Pyrexia
- BP: hypotension is a sign of systemic sepsis and warrants immediate medical assistance
- O_2 saturation via pulse oximetry

Key investigations
- CXR: involvement of >one lobe is associated with a poorer prognosis
- ABGs
- FBC, U&Es, CRP
- 12-lead ECG

Key actions and treatment
- Check airway, breathing, and circulation
- Regular recordings of vital signs
- Give high-flow O_2 initially and review following blood gas analysis
- IV access and IV fluids if dehydrated
- Paracetamol (oral or IV) to reduce pyrexia
- Antibiotics (oral or IV): see local guidelines
- Nurse patient in an upright position if possible: this will improve ventilation

① Anaemia

Anaemia is the end result of several conditions which cause the number of red blood cells to decrease, which reduces the O_2 carrying capacity of the blood. In order to provide adequate tissue oxygenation, the heart and lungs have to work harder resulting, amongst other symptoms, in dyspnoea.

Key signs and symptoms
- Dyspnoea
- Tiredness/lack of energy
- Palpitations
- Lightheadedness
- Pallor
- Angina

Key history and assessment
- Heavy periods: menorrhagia
- Poor diet
- GI bleeding: melaena
- Blood disorders—e.g. leukaemia
- Drug history: aspirin and steroids increase the risk of GI bleeding

Key observations and findings
- Respiratory rate: may be elevated
- O_2 saturation: usually normal
- Pulse: may be tachycardic in severe cases
- BP: usually normal
- Temperature

Key investigations
- FBC
- Vitamin B12, and folic acid levels
- Group and cross match if necessary

Key actions and treatment
- High-flow O_2 if symptoms of shortness of breath are severe
- Referral for medical assessment

① Malignancy

Patients with bronchial carcinoma may experience dyspnoea. This may be the first presentation of the disease or patients with an established diagnosis may attend for emergency care if their condition deteriorates acutely.

Key signs and symptoms
- Increasing dyspnoea
- Haemoptysis
- Fatigue
- Anorexia/weight loss
- Persistent cough

Key history and assessment
- Known diagnosis of bronchial carcinoma
- Recent weight loss
- Loss of appetite
- Chest infection which has failed to resolve with treatment
- Smoking

Key observations and findings
- Tachycardia
- Tachypnoea and dyspnoea
- O_2 saturation
- BP: usually normal
- Temperature

Key investigations
- CXR
- Blood for FBC and U&Es

Key actions and treatment
- High-flow O_2 via non-rebreathing mask
- IV access for pain relief if required
- Medical referral for investigation and management

Sore throat

Differential diagnosis

:◉: True emergencies
- Epiglottitis
- Ingestion of caustic substance
- Obstructed airway

:◎: Urgent presentations
- Foreign body
- Ludwig's angina
- Peritonsillar abscess (quinsy)

① Timely assessment
- Postoperative problems

⑦ Non-urgent presentations
- Mumps
- Tonsillitis
- Upper respiratory tract infection

Introduction

Sore throat is a very common complaint. Most patients will present to their GP; however, some will attend emergency departments or other healthcare providers. Most patients will have a simple URTI.

However, there are some conditions which may progress rapidly, leading to airway obstruction which requires immediate intervention by experienced specialist teams. It is important to recognize these conditions and expedite the transfer of these patients to the appropriate clinical setting as rapidly as possible.

☠ Epiglottitis

Infection of the epiglottis was once principally a childhood illness caused by *Haemophilus influenzae* type B. However, following the introduction of the HIB vaccination programme, childhood epiglottitis has become much less common. The condition can also occur in adults as a result of streptococcal or staphylococcal infection. Epiglottitis is a potentially life-threatening condition and senior medical help must be obtained immediately. If the condition is suspected from the patient's symptoms *do not examine the throat* as this can precipitate airway obstruction.

Key signs and symptoms
- Pyrexia
- Stridor
- Dysphagia
- Drooling of saliva
- Hoarse voice
- Symptoms partially relieved by sitting up and leaning forward

Key history and assessment
- *This is a life-threatening condition*
- The presence of stridor and pyrexia should alert the practitioner to the possibility of epiglottitis
- As soon as epiglottitis is suspected senior medical help must be sought at once. In a community setting ambulance transfer of the patient to a unit with full resuscitation facilities must be arranged as soon as possible.
- *Do not examine the mouth or throat until an experienced anaesthetist is present*

Key observations
- Do not delay obtaining senior medical help if epiglottis is suspected by undertaking observations
- Pyrexia: >38.5°C
- Tachycardia
- Tachypnoea
- Stridor
- O_2 saturation: if <94% significant airway obstruction is likely to be present
- BP: likely to be normal until patient is in extremis, then hypotensive

Key investigations
- Do not delay obtaining senior medical help by undertaking investigations. The stress caused by venepuncture may be sufficient to precipitate airway obstruction.

Key actions and treatment
- Obtain senior medical help immediately, in a community setting request an emergency ambulance
- Do not examine the throat due to the risk of causing complete airway obstruction
- Emergency referral to an experienced anaesthetist and/or ENT specialist
- Give humidified O_2
- 5mg nebulized adrenaline may provide temporary relief
- Allow the patient to remain in a position which provides them with the greatest comfort, usually upright and leaning forward
- Prepare equipment for intubation if available

☠: **Ingestion of caustic substance**

Caustic substances may be ingested accidentally or deliberately and cause direct injury to the throat, oesophagus, and stomach. In addition, injury to the airways may occur through inhalation or aspiration of chemicals.

Key signs and symptoms
- Evidence of airway injury—e.g. stridor, wheeze, dyspnoea
- Hoarseness
- Coughing
- Burns/blistering to the mouth and lips
- Vomiting
- Dysphagia

Key history and assessment
- Identify nature and quantity of substance ingested if possible
- Accidental or intentional ingestion?

Key observations and findings
- Respiratory rate:
  - tachypnoea
  - dyspnoea
  - stridor indicates upper airway injury
  - wheeze may indicate lower airway injury
- Pulse: tachycardia
- BP

Key investigations
- ABG
- CXR: may indicate pulmonary injury

Key actions and treatment
- Take appropriate action to avoid self-contamination
- Refer to anaesthetist for airway assessment and management
- Obtain information about the substance ingested; this may involve contacting the manufacturer or Poisons Information Service—follow the instructions regarding treatment

☠ Obstructed airway

Regardless of the underlying cause patients presenting with a sore throat who are experiencing airway or breathing difficulties require assessment by a senior doctor immediately, preferably an anaesthetist.

Key signs and symptoms

- Distressed patient
- Dyspnoea
- Stridor: a high-pitch sound which is worse on inspiration
- Tachypnoea progressing, as the patient becomes fatigued, to bradyp-noea and respiratory arrest
- Cyanosis

Key history and assessment

- *Do not examine the mouth or throat until an experienced anaesthetist is present*—risk of precipitating complete obstruction

Key observations and findings

- Do not delay referral to undertake observations
- Respiratory rate:
  - tachypnoea is common
  - bradypnoea indicates imminent respiratory arrest and is a clinical emergency
- O_2 saturation: <94% indicates significant airway obstruction
- Pulse:
  - tachycardia
  - bradycardia is a sign of a patient *in extremis*
- BP
- Cardiac monitoring
- Temperature: pyrexia may indicate infection

Key investigations

- No invasive tests should be performed until the airway has been assessed and secured if necessary

Key actions and treatment

- Emergency referral to a senior anaesthetist and/or ENT specialist
- Give 100% humidified O_2
- 5mg nebulized adrenaline may provide temporary relief
- Allow the patient to adopt any position in which they are comfortable
- Prepare equipment for intubation if required

:⚙: Foreign body

The most common causes of a retained FB in the throat/upper oesophagus are a food bolus or fish/chicken bone. If there is any indication of airway obstruction immediate assessment by an anaesthetist is required. If the patient is distressed and cannot swallow his/her own saliva then an urgent ENT assessment is required. In the presence of pyrexia other conditions such as epiglottitis or quinsy should be considered.

📖 See Foreign bodies, p.233.

:⚙: Ludwig's angina

Ludwig's angina is rare and results from a bilateral cellulitis of the submandibular, sublingual, and submental spaces which progresses rapidly causing gross swelling of the neck and mouth. It is a potential airway emergency with a mortality rate of 75% if not treated rapidly.

Key signs and symptoms
- Massive, tense swelling bilaterally in the neck
- Systemically unwell with pyrexia and tachycardia
- Swelling of the floor of the mouth forcing the tongue upwards
- Difficulty in breathing, swallowing, and talking
- Inability to protrude the tongue
- Hypoxia

Key history and assessment
- Infected dental caries
- Recent trauma resulting in mandibular fractures

Key observations
- Respiratory rate
- Pulse oximetry
- Pulse
- Cardiac monitoring
- BP
- Temperature

Key actions and treatment
- Emergency referral to anaesthetics and ENT
- Maintain the airway if necessary
- Give high concentration of humidified O_2
- IV access
- IV antibiotics and fluids according to local guidelines
- Continuous monitoring of vital signs

:☼: Peritonsillar abscess (quinsy)

Quinsy results from the spread of infection from the tonsils into the nearby soft tissues resulting in a unilateral swelling which may be large enough to displace the uvula. The patient presents with sore throat, dysphasia, and fever.

Key signs and symptoms
- Sore throat: often unilateral
- Fever
- Dysphagia
- Dehydration
- Trismus—inability to open mouth due to spasm of the masseter muscles
- Uvula displaced by peritonsillar swelling
- Enlarged cervical lymph nodes

Key history and assessment
- Recent tonsillitis
- Worsening fever
- Dysphagia

Key observations and findings
- Respiratory rate: tachypnoea
- Pulse: tachycardia
- O_2 saturation should be recorded
- BP should be recorded
- Temperature: pyrexia is usual

Key investigations
- None normally required

Key actions and treatment
- Urgent referral to ENT team for aspiration or drainage
- IV cannula and antibiotics according to local guidelines
- IV fluids may be required
- Analgesia as required

① Postoperative problems

Patients with postoperative problems following throat surgery may present for emergency care. Presenting problems include pain, infection, or bleeding. Post-tonsillectomy bleeding can be severe and may be underestimated. Significant haemorrhage should be managed with IV fluids/blood transfusion as necessary. Analgesia should be provided as required. Following initial management the patient should be referred to the ENT surgeons for definitive care.

② Mumps

The frequency of mumps has dropped substantially following the introduction of MMR vaccination programmes. The incubation period of the disease is 14–21 days prior to the onset of symptoms which consist of fever, malaise, and painful, swollen, parotid glands. Symptoms normally last around 14 days followed by a full recovery. The main complications of mumps (hearing loss and male sterility) are rare. Treatment is conservative and primarily involves maintaining patient comfort.

⑦ Tonsillitis

Acute tonsillitis may be viral or bacterial in origin. The tonsils become swollen and painful with pustules forming if the condition is bacterial in nature.

Key signs and symptoms
- Sore throat
- Fever
- Headache
- Mild dysphagia

Key history and assessment
- Previous history of tonsillitis

Key observations and findings
- Swelling of the tonsils
- Presence of pus on the tonsils
- Pyrexia
- Enlarged cervical lymph nodes

Key investigations
- None usually required

Key actions and treatment
- Where a bacterial infection is suspected antibiotics are required: see local guidelines
- Viral infections are treated symptomatically with paracetamol

⑦ Upper respiratory tract infection

URTI is a common cause of a mild sore throat. The condition is viral in origin and is self-limiting. Supportive treatment only is required.

Further reading

Perry M (2005). *Head, Neck and Dental Emergencies.* Oxford: Oxford University Press.

Testicular pain

Differential diagnosis

True emergencies
- Testicular torsion

Urgent presentations
- Trauma

Non-urgent presentations
- Epididymo-orchitis
- Hydrocele

Introduction

Testicular pain is a surgical emergency until torsion has been excluded. Testicular pain is often severe and may be combined with anxiety and embarrassment; tact and privacy should therefore be maintained at all times.

☠ Testicular torsion

Testicular torsion occurs where the spermatic cord becomes twisted causing compression, amongst other things, of the blood vessels supplying the testis. The condition often occurs where there is a congenital problem such as a maldescended testis. If untreated the resulting testicular hypoxia will result in permanent damage and possible infertility. As such, torsion is a surgical emergency and referral should occur as soon as the condition is suspected.

Key signs and symptoms
- Sudden onset of severe unilateral pain
- Pain may radiate into the abdomen
- N&V

Key history and assessment
- History of congenital testicular problems or previous torsion
- Diagnosis based of assessment of pain and onset of symptoms
- The condition is most common up to the age of 20

Key observations and findings
- Pulse: tachycardia due to pain and anxiety
- BP: may be raised due to pain
- Respiratory rate: should be normal
- Temperature: normal
- Extremely painful testis on palpation
- Unilateral swollen testis

Key investigations
- Diagnosis made on clinical assessment

Key actions and treatment
- Analgesia: normally IV
- Keep nil-by-mouth
- Refer for urgent surgical assessment

:✿: Trauma

Trauma to the testes may involve blunt trauma, lacerations, or testicular rupture. Pain is severe and may radiate to the abdomen. The patient often experiences N&V.

Key signs and symptoms
- Obvious scrotal injury
- Pallor, nausea, vomiting

Key history and assessment
- Obtain mechanism of injury from patient
- Consideration should be given to the possibility of abuse where the history and/or mechanism of injury seems inappropriate

Key observations and findings
- Obvious scrotal injury: laceration, swelling, haematoma
- If swelling is unilateral consider torsion

Key investigations
- Urinalysis for blood to exclude urethral injury
- Ultrasound examination (organized by physician) may help in diagnosing significant injuries

Key actions and treatment
- Analgesia
- Manage wounds as appropriate
- If torsion is suspected or a large haematoma/laceration is present refer for surgical assessment

⑦ Epididymo-orchitis

Epididymo-orchitis describes an infection of the testes and spermatic cord. In younger adults the condition often results from chlamydial or gonorrheal infection. In the elderly it occurs more commonly following a UTI.

Key signs and symptoms
- Unilateral testicular pain, gradual in onset
- Red, inflamed scrotum, may be localized to one side
- Dysuria
- Urethral discharge may be present if the causative agent is a STD

Key history and assessment
- Gradual onset of symptoms
- History of chlamydial or gonorrheal infection
- Recent UTI
- Lifting the scrotum may ease the pain: Prehn's sign

Key observations and findings
- Temperature: pyrexia may be present
- Pulse: usually normal
- BP: should be normal

Key investigations
- Urinalysis
- Urine for C&S
- Urethral swab if discharge present

Key actions and treatment
- Analgesia, NSAID
- Antibiotic therapy according to local guidelines
- The condition may be difficult to differentiate from torsion. If urinalysis is negative obtain an urgent surgical assessment
- Referral to genitourinary medicine if suspected STD

⑦ Hydrocele

Hydrocele is a painless swelling of the scrotum as a result of fluid accumulation around one or both testes. They rarely present as emergencies and no urgent treatment is required. Referral to primary care is appropriate.

Torso injury

Differential diagnosis

:۞: **True emergencies**

- Aortic rupture
- Cardiac tamponade
- Flail chest
- Gastrointestinal tract injuries
- Haemothorax
- Pelvic fractures
- Pulmonary contusion

:۞: **Urgent presentations**

- Bladder and urethra injury
- Hepatic injury
- Myocardial contusion
- Obvious open wound
- Pancreatic injury
- Pneumothorax
- Renal trauma
- Rib fractures
- Splenic injury
- Sternal fractures

Introduction

Organs within the torso may be damaged by blunt or penetrating trauma. In the setting of trauma it is important to remember that several organs in different compartments may be injured.

The management of patients with torso injuries should, like all major trauma, follow the principles of airway, breathing, circulation. Signs of respiratory distress or cardiovascular instability require immediate medical attention and early anaesthetics involvement.

External injuries (particularly penetrating wounds) may appear innocuous and mask significant internal injuries. Injuries to the back are easily overlooked when the patient is lying prone. It is therefore important to remember to perform a log roll and examine the patient's back to exclude these injuries.

Assessment of the chest should include checking for:
- Obvious deformities
- Open wounds
- Unequal chest movement
- Tenderness
- Crepitations on palpation: surgical emphysema
- Equal breath sounds

Abdominal and pelvic assessment should be focused on identifying and managing haemorrhage or peritoneal contamination. If the patient is haemodynamically unstable this must be addressed prior to determining an exact diagnosis.

:☠: Aortic rupture

Survival rates from traumatic rupture of the aorta are extremely low with the vast majority of victims dying at the scene. The mechanism of injury is a shearing force which tears the vessel wall resulting in catastrophic haemorrhage.

If the patient survives the journey to hospital he/she is likely to be haemodynamically compromised, and will commonly have other major chest injuries. Management will follow the principles of ATLS and usually involves a trauma team.

📖 See Major trauma, p.293.

:☼: Cardiac tamponade

Bleeding into the pericardial sac may occur following blunt or penetrating trauma. This may cause compression of the heart muscle which, if severe, can compromise cardiac output. If the condition is not resolved rapidly, cardiac arrest may occur.

Key signs and symptoms
- Signs of cardiac tamponade may be subtle
- Evidence of chest trauma
- Chest pain which may be exacerbated by breathing
- Shortness of breath
- Cyanosis
- Altered conscious level

Key history and assessment
- History of recent significant trauma—e.g. road traffic collision, stab wound
- Cardiac injury should be excluded in all patients with chest or epigastric injuries
- Pneumothorax should be excluded
- Presence of shock not responding to fluid resuscitation

Key observations and findings
- Tachypnoea
- Tachycardia: peripheral pulses may be weak or absent
- Hypotension
- SpO_2: may be <94%

Key investigations
- FAST scan if available
- 12-lead ECG abnormalities are common and are not diagnostic
- Echocardiogram is required if available
- FBC, U&Es, ABGs

Key actions and treatment
- Immediate senior medical intervention required
- Manage airway breathing and circulation
- High-flow O_2 via a non-rebreathing mask
- IV access
- IV fluids
- Cardiac monitoring required
- Pericardiocentesis may relieve the pericardial pressure and can be life saving
- Emergency thoracotomy will be required as soon as possible

:☹: Flail chest

A flail chest occurs where several ribs are fractured in more than one place. This creates a 'floating' chest wall segment which moves in the wrong direction when the patient breathes. This compromises respiration and is often associated with significant underlying lung injuries such as pulmonary contusion or pneumothorax. These patients are seriously injured and usually require transfer to HDU/ITU following stabilization in the emergency department.

Key signs and symptoms
- Paradoxical rib movements
- Dyspnoea
- Severe chest wall pain
- Evidence of chest wall injury

Key history and assessment
- Diagnosis based on mechanism of injury and presence of paradoxical chest wall movement
- Crepitation on palpation

Key observations and findings
- Tachypnoea
- Poor chest wall expansion due to pain
- Paradoxical chest wall movement
- Tachycardia
- BP: hypotension may indicate underlying haemorrhage
- SpO_2: if <94% will require further assessment and respiratory support

Key investigations
- Clinical diagnosis made following observation of chest wall movement
- CXR to confirm rib fractures and underlying lung damage, haemothorax, or pneumothorax
- 12-lead ECG for arrhythmias
- FBC, U&Es, group and save, ABGs
- A CT of the chest will provide a more accurate clinical picture, but should only be performed once the patient has been stabilized

Key actions and treatment
- Immediate medical assessment and involvement of senior clinician
- High-flow O_2 via a non-rebreathing mask
- Stabilize flail segment with local direct pressure
- Cardiac monitoring
- IV access × 2
- IV fluids as required
- IV analgesia titrated to effect
- Urgent anaesthetics opinion required

☣ Gastrointestinal tract injuries

As with chest trauma, GI tract injuries may result from blunt or penetrating trauma. In addition to the risk of haemorrhage, rupture of the gut carries the risk of peritoneal contamination and subsequent life-threatening infection.

Key signs and symptoms
- Evidence of external abdominal wall injury: posterior abdominal wall injuries should be excluded during the log roll procedure
- Pain: dependent on the site of injury—may radiate to the shoulder
- Signs of haemorrhage: tachycardia, hypotension
- Signs of peritonitis:
  - rigid, tender abdomen
  - N&V

Key history and assessment
- History of significant mechanism of injury

Key observations and findings
- Tachypnoea
- Tachycardia
- BP: hypotension may result from haemorrhage (early) or sepsis (late)
- Pyrexia suggests infection

Key investigations
- Ultrasound (FAST scan) will identify the presence of free blood in the peritoneal cavity
- FBC, U&Es, group and save/cross-match as required
- Urinalysis: frank haematuria indicates renal injuries
- CT scan may provide a more accurate clinical picture once the patient has been stabilized

Key actions and treatment
- Senior ED and surgical assessment required
- High-flow O_2 via a non-rebreathing mask
- IV access × 2
- IV fluids
- IV analgesia
- Definitive treatment will depend on the patient's condition and on the findings of the investigations

☠ Haemothorax

The signs and symptoms of a haemothorax and the treatment required will depend on the severity of the haemorrhage and associated injuries to the major organs within the chest cavity.

Key signs and symptoms
- Evidence of chest wall trauma
- Dyspnoea
- Tachypnoea
- Tachycardia

Key history and assessment
- Significant mechanism of injury
- Check for tracheal deviation: may occur with tension pneumothorax or major haemorrhage
- Decreased breath sounds on affected side
- Dullness to percussion

Key observations and findings
- Dyspnoea and tachypnoea
- SpO_2 may be low
- Tachycardia
- Hypotension due to blood loss

Key investigations
- CXR: upright if possible—supine films may fail to demonstrate a haemothorax
- FBC, U&Es, ABGs, group and save/cross match as required
- CT if patient is stable

Key actions and treatment
- Urgent senior ED review
- High flow O_2 via a non-rebreathing mask
- IV access
- IV fluids
- ECG monitoring
- IV analgesia
- Intercostal drain required

:Ö: Pelvic fractures

Pelvic fractures occur as a result of significant blunt trauma and can be associated with major haemorrhage. The exception to this rule is a fracture to the pubic rami resulting from minimal trauma following a fall in the elderly or osteoporotic patient. These injuries are not associated with significant bleeding and require analgesia and active mobilization.

Key signs and symptoms
- Pain on movement or palpation of pelvis
- Crepitus
- Inability to straight leg raise
- Tachycardia
- Hypotension

Key history and assessment
- Mechanism of injury
- Signs of hypovolaemia
- Other associated injuries
- Bruising to the scrotum or buttocks
- PV bleeding
- Bleeding from external urethral meatus
- Assess lower limbs for paraesthesia

Key observations and findings
- Tachypnoea: may indicate hypovolaemia
- Tachycardia: may indicate hypovolaemia or pain
- BP: hypotension suggests severe blood loss and requires fluid resuscitation

Key investigations
- Pelvic XR
- Other XRs as required to exclude associated injuries
- FBC, U&Es, group and cross match if signs of hypovolaemia

Key actions and treatment
- Senior ED and orthopaedic review required unless isolated pubic rami fractures
- IV access × 2
- IV fluid and blood transfusion as required
- IV analgesia
- Immobilization using a sheet or alternative device is required for unstable fractures to reduce haemorrhage
- Isolated pubic rami fractures require analgesia and gradual mobilization

☠ Pulmonary contusion

Blunt trauma to the chest wall may result in bruising to the underlying lung. This injury is dynamic in nature and the patient commonly deteriorates over the ensuing 6–12 hours.

Key signs and symptoms
- Initial signs and symptoms may be mild
- Bruising to chest wall
- Signs of respiratory distress indicate a serious injury and require immediate medical attention

Key history and assessment
- Mechanism of injury
- Difficult to determine on physical examination
- Crackles may be present on auscultation

Key observations and findings
- Tachypnoea and dyspnoea indicate a significant injury
- SpO_2: <94% suggests a significant injury
- Tachycardia: due to respiratory distress and pain
- BP: should be normal. Hypotension suggests the patient has a significant haemorrhage

Key investigations
- CXR
- CT chest: provided the patient is stable
- ABGs, FBC, U&E, group and save: as these patients often have associated injuries

Key actions and treatment
- Urgent senior medical assessment required
- Early ITU review if the patient has respiratory distress
- High-flow O_2 with non-rebreathing mask
- IV access × 2
- IV fluid if patient shows signs of hypovolaemia
- IV analgesia
- Most patients will require management in a HDU/ICU

☠ Bladder and urethra injury

The bladder may be injured following blunt or penetrating trauma. In particular, damage to the urethra may result from a pelvic fracture.

Key signs and symptoms
- Haematuria
- Bleeding from the urethral meatus
- Suprapubic pain
- Perineal haematoma
- Scrotal haematoma
- Inability to pass urine

Key history and assessment
- Mechanism of injury
- History of blunt or penetrating trauma

Key observations and findings
- Monitor respirations, pulse, BP and temperature; any abnormalities require further assessment and appropriate management.
- Presence of pelvic fracture increases risks of urethral injury
- Rectal examination (by a physician): high-riding prostate indicate urethral rupture

Key investigations
- Pelvic XR
- If injuries to the urethra are suspected, contrast studies are required

Key actions and treatment
- Urgent medical assessment/intervention required
- Assess and manage ABC
- Secure IV access and withdraw blood for group and hold/cross match as appropriate
- IV fluids/blood transfusion as required
- Analgesia as required
- Do not pass a urinary catheter until urethral injury has been excluded

☼ Hepatic injury

Laceration to the liver can occur following both blunt and penetrating trauma and can result in life-threatening haemorrhage.

Key signs and symptoms
- Evidence of abdominal/chest wall trauma
- Abdominal pain: generalized or right upper quadrant
- N&V
- Signs of hypovolaemia

Key history and assessment
- Significant mechanism of injury
- Presence of lower rib fractures on the right side
- Penetrating trauma to abdomen or lower chest wall

Key observations and findings
- Tachypnoea: due to hypovolaemia and/or pain
- Tachycardia: due to blood loss
- Hypotension: due to hypovolaemia
- Abdominal wall tenderness in the right upper quadrant or generally

Key investigations
- Ultrasound: FAST scan
- Abdominal CT scan: provided the patient is stable
- FBC, U&E, group and cross match as required

Key actions and treatment
- Senior ED review required
- High-flow O_2 via a non-rebreathing mask
- IV access × 2
- IV fluid as required
- IV analgesia
- The majority of patients are treated conservatively

☼ Myocardial contusion

Bruising of the myocardium occurs most commonly following blunt trauma.
It may be asymptomatic or it may result in life-threatening arrhythmias.

Key signs and symptoms
- Evidence of chest wall injury
- Chest pain

Key history and assessment
- Deceleration injury is the most common mechanism

Key observations and findings
- Tachycardia unrelated to haemorrhage
- Tachypnoea may be present
- BP usually normal unless significant arrhythmia is present

Key investigations
- 12-lead ECG: may be normal or ST elevation—this does *not* indicate ischaemia
- FBC, U&E ABGs, cardiac enzymes
- XR: to exclude other chest injuries
- Echocardiogram: will identify abnormal cardiac motion and pericardial bleeding

Key actions and treatment
- Urgent senior ED review required
- Give high-flow O_2 via a non-rebreathing mask
- Cardiac monitoring
- IV access
- Analgesia as required for associated chest wall injuries
- Treat arrhythmias as appropriate

☼ Obvious open wound

Chest wound

Open wounds to the chest wall may cause a pneumothorax which may result from air entry through the wound and/or air exit from an injury to the underlying lung. Open wounds should be covered with an occlusive dressing *taped on three sides* which allows air to escape on expiration, whilst preventing air entry on inspiration. The patient will need a chest drain inserted as soon as possible.

Abdominal wound

Open abdominal wounds should be covered with a sterile dressing as quickly as possible to prevent contamination. Warm saline packs can be used and covered with a low adherent dressing which can be removed without causing further trauma. If the wound is larger than the available dressings, cling film or the wrapping from any sterile pack, placed inner surface towards the wound may be used. Abdominal contents which have herniated through the wound should not be replaced. Immediate surgical referral is required.

☼ Pancreatic injury

Injury to the pancreas usually occurs following blunt trauma to the abdomen and is often accompanied by hepatic or bowel injury. The patient experiences abdominal pain which may radiate to the back and shoulder. Surgical referral is required for ongoing monitoring, assessment, and management.

☼ Pneumothorax

Traumatic pneumothorax can occur following blunt or penetrating trauma. The presence of air in the pleural space prevents the lungs from fully expanding. The presence of a tension pneumothorax in which the chest contents are deviated to one side is a life-threatening emergency which requires immediate intervention.

📖 See Shortness of breath, p.367.

☼ Renal trauma

Blunt trauma is the most common cause of renal injuries. Bleeding occurs into the retro-peritoneal space and cannot be detected by FAST scanning or diagnostic peritoneal lavage (DPL).

Key signs and symptoms
- Loin pain.
- Lower rib fractures
- Frank haematuria

Key history and assessment
- Frank haematuria is the most obvious sign of renal injury
- Exclude other abdominal injuries, as isolated renal injuries are unusual
- Tachycardia and hypotension suggests significant bleeding

Key observations and findings
- Vital signs may initially be normal: continued monitoring required
- Tachypnoea, tachycardia and hypotension suggest significant haemorrhage

Key investigations
- CT scan is the investigation of choice
- Ultrasound may be a safer investigation in the unstable patient
- Urinalysis
- FBC, U&E, group and save/cross match as required

Key actions and treatment
- Urgent senior ED assessment
- IV access
- IV fluids as required
- IV analgesia
- Most patient can be managed conservatively

☼ Rib fractures

Patients presenting with rib fractures are common in the emergency department. These are mostly minor injuries, requiring simple analgesia. However, care should be taken to exclude more serious injuries such as flail chest or pulmonary contusion, particularly following a significant mechanism of injury as such as a road traffic collision.

Key signs and symptoms
- Chest wall bruising
- Pain on breathing or coughing

Key history and assessment
- Mechanism of injury and force involved
- Signs of respiratory distress suggests significant associated injury
- Pre-existing respiratory disease: patient with COPD are more likely to require in-patient management

Key observations and findings
- Dyspnoea: may occur due to pain or other significant injuries
- Tachycardia: may occur due to pain or other significant injuries
- SpO$_2$: should be normal

Key investigations
- CXR
- ABGs: if patient is showing signs of respiratory distress

Key actions and treatment
- Patient with no respiratory embarrassment may be discharged if pain is adequately controlled and the patient can self-care
- Encourage deep breathing and coughing
- Advise the patient that pain will persist for 1–2 weeks
- Patients with respiratory distress and/or multiple fractures require:
  • senior ED review
  • high-flow O$_2$ by non-rebreathing mask
  • admission for pain control and physiotherapy

☼ Splenic injury

The spleen is commonly injured in blunt abdominal trauma. Patients may present acutely or they can have a delayed presentation. One of the commonest mechanisms of injury is a fall from a bicycle with the handlebar striking the left upper quadrant. Fractures of the lower ribs on the left should raise suspicion of this injury, as should evidence of unexplained blood loss. The spleen is the most vascular organ in the body and injuries can result in severe blood loss.

Key signs and symptoms
- Initial signs of injury may be subtle or absent
- Abdominal pain in the upper left quadrant
- Left shoulder pain may be present
- Signs of hypovolaemia

Key history and assessment
- History of trauma which may seem minor
- Left upper quadrant bruising/pain

Key observations and findings
- Initial vital signs may appear normal
- If splenic injury is suspected monitoring of vital signs is required
- Tachypnoea, tachycardia, hypotension suggests hypovolaemia

Key investigations
- If hypovolaemia is present the patient requires resuscitation followed by urgent surgical review
- Abdominal CT scanning is the investigation of choice provided the patient is stable
- Ultrasound may identify free abdominal fluid (blood)
- FBC, U&E, group and save or cross match as appropriate

Key actions and treatment
- Urgent senior ED assessment required
- High-flow O_2 via a non re-breathing mask
- Continuous vital signs and cardiac monitoring
- IV access × 2
- Fluid resuscitation as required
- IV analgesia
- Admit for monitoring and surgical intervention as appropriate

:⚙: **Sternal fractures**

Sternum fractures most commonly occur as a result of seatbelt trauma. Often the fracture involves the outer cortex only and can be managed with simple analgesia. Provided there are no other significant injuries the patient can be discharged.

Urinary problems

Differential diagnosis

:☼: **Urgent presentations**
- Priapism
- Trauma
- Urinary retention

① **Timely assessment**
- Urinary tract infection

⑦ **Non urgent presentation**
- Sexually transmitted diseases

Introduction

Most patients with urinary problems present with obstruction/hesitation, dysuria (pain on micturition), or frank haematuria (blood in the urine). Haematuria may occur in patients who have a severe case of cystitis (haemorrhagic cystitis), pyelonephritis, or following trauma to the abdomen, where frank haematuria may result from injury to the kidney. In the latter, a CT scan of the abdomen may be required in order to identify the severity of the renal injury and other associated injuries to the abdominal contents.

⚙ Priapism

Priapism is a penile erection which is not associated with sexual stimulation and causes discomfort for the patient. Priapism may be spontaneous or iatrogenic (as a result of treatment for erectile dysfunction). History of taking sildenafil (Viagra®) should be specifically sought. In the setting of trauma, priapism may occur where the patient has suffered cervical cord damage following, for example, a road traffic collision.

Key signs and symptoms
- Penile erection

Key history and assessment
- Trauma
- Injection of prostaglandins for erectile dysfunction
- Time of onset

Key observation and findings
- Vital signs should be normal

Key investigations
- None required

Key actions and treatments
- In the setting of trauma appropriate trauma management guidelines should be followed
- Urgent referral to urologist for assessment and management

:⚙: Trauma

Trauma can occur to any part of the urinary tract. It is more common in males resulting either from isolated injuries or as part of multiple trauma.

Key signs and symptoms
- Blood from the urethral meatus
- Perineal bruising
- Inability to void urine

Key history and assessment
- Consider the mechanism of injury and potential injury patterns
- High-riding prostate on rectal examination

Key observation and findings
- Vital signs should be normal: abnormalities should raise concern regarding significant associated injuries

Key investigations
- Depend on the nature and extent of the trauma

Key actions and treatments
- Do not pass urethral catheter
- Following stabilization if necessary, referral to general surgeon or urologist for further management

:⊕: **Urinary retention**

The inability to voluntarily fully empty the bladder occurs most commonly in older males. Emergency presentation is due to pain and discomfort.

Key signs and symptoms
- Inability to void urine
- Suprapubic pain due to enlarged bladder

Key history and assessment
- Palpable bladder
- History of prostate problems
- History of UTI

Key observations and findings
- Vital signs should be normal

Key investigations
- None required initially

Key actions and treatment
- Urethral catheterization at the earliest opportunity
- If unable to pass urethral catheter consider suprapubic catheter
- Consider referral to urology for investigation
- Following successful drainage of bladder, the patient may be discharged with follow-up in the community

① Urinary tract infection

Urinary tract infections can affect either the upper urinary tract (pyelone-phritis) or the lower urinary tract (cystitis or urethritis).

Cystitis

Infection of the bladder (cystitis) is more common in females. The condition presents with dysuria and urinary frequency. Treatment is normally straightforward with oral fluids and antibiotics (see local guidelines). Prior to treatment a sample of urine should be sent for C&S. It is always worth checking the patients blood glucose in order to detect previously undiagnosed diabetes. Most patients can be managed in the community with primary care follow-up.

Pyelonephritis

Kidney infection (pyelonephritis) results from a bacterial infection and is more common in younger patients. Patients typically present with fever, malaise, and loin pain on the affected side. Dysuria is not normally present. Patients can be managed with simple analgesics, fluids, and antibiotics according to local guidelines. If the patient is well enough they may be discharged with primary care follow-up. If, however, the patient is systemically unwell he/she may require admission for IV fluids and antibiotics. As for cystitis, urine should be sent for C&S prior to treatment and the patients blood glucose should be checked.

Urethritis

Infection of the urethra (urethritis) is usually bacterial, with *Escherichia coli* being the commonest cause. The condition is particularly common in females. Urethritis presents with dysuria and malaise. Patients are normally treated with simple analgesia, oral fluids, and antibiotics according to local guidelines. Once again urine should be sent for C&S and blood glucose checked.

⑦ Sexually transmitted diseases

A number of STDs can present for emergency care with urinary symptoms. It is important to be aware that patients may have more than one STD therefore a full medical history, sexual health history, and HIV status (if known to the patient) should be obtained. Once STD is suspected treatment, investigation and ongoing management is more appropriately undertaken in a GUM clinic.

Wounds

Differential diagnosis

True emergencies
- Major haemorrhage
- Gunshot wounds
- Stab wounds

Timely assessment
- Minor haemorrhage

Principles of wound care

Regardless of the site and severity of wounds there are a number of over-riding principles in traumatic wound care.

Cleaning

Traumatic wounds must be considered contaminated and therefore require through cleaning. The most effective method is by irrigation with tap water or saline. Gross contamination can be removed with liquid soap. Oil- or grease-based contamination can be removed with commercially available degreasers. All cleaning products used should be removed by copious irrigation. Debridement, if necessary, can be performed under LA or GA. Wounds should be carefully explored and all necrotic or devitalized tissues removed. For abrasions it is not always possible to completely remove all the contaminants. It is therefore worth considering the use of hydrogels covered with a film dressing to help bring foreign material to the surface. The alternative is gentle brushing with a soft toothbrush to remove loose material. This is effective but can be painful.

Wound types and suitable dressings

Wounds should be thoroughly clean and dry and haemostasis achieved before a dressing is considered. The dressing should be appropriate to the anatomical site and stage of healing. It should also be comfortable and acceptable to the patient. If the patient is to be discharged, written wound care advice should always be given. This should include any referral for follow up if required and information regarding indications for seeking further health care advice. Ensure the patient understands this, and indications for seeking any further health care input.

Abrasions

Abrasions (grazes) are superficial wounds which do not penetrate the full thickness of the skin. Despite this they are often extremely painful. After thorough cleaning they may be left exposed or covered with a film dressing to reduce the risk of secondary infection. If the wound is oozing this can be controlled with an alginate, foam, hydrocellular, hydrocolloid, or sheet gel dressing.

Bites

Bite wounds have a high infection risk due to contamination and deep penetration. The risk is greatest following human bites. All bite wounds should be thoroughly irrigated. Where the wound is close to a joint or has penetrated deeply (in particular in the hand) oral antibiotics should be considered. Suturing should be avoided as this may encourage infection and abscess formation.

Crush injuries

Crush injuries are often associated with severe tissue damage and devitalization. There may be associated underlying injuries such as fractures which may require a specialist opinion. Subungual haematomas following a crush to a finger tip can be released by trephining the nail.

Degloving injuries

Degloving wounds result from shearing injuries which result in layers of tissues being torn away, often exposing deeper anatomical structures. These wounds require an urgent medical review and surgery is often required. Initial dressings must be low- or non-adherent. Cling film is often the best choice and may be covered with padding and bandages.

Lacerations

After thorough exploration to ensure no underlying structures are damaged, no FBs are present and the wound is clean, primary closure (using LA) should be undertaken. Sutures, staples, adhesive strips, or tissue adhesive may be used depending on the individual wound. Dressings should be low/non-adherent, but in the presence of exudate may also need to be absorbent. Pressure dressings may also be required. Do not overlook the humble sticking plaster for simple lacerations.

Penetrating wounds

The treatment of penetrating injuries depends on the mechanism of injury involved. Large objects such as knives should not be removed in the emergency setting as further injury or uncontrollable haemorrhage may result. Minor penetrating injuries (puncture wounds) can be treated by removing the object, cleaning, and dressing the wound after confirming there is no underlying tendon or neurovascular damage. In cases of assault resulting in penetrating wounds consideration should be given to the legal requirements of reporting serious assaults and the handling of evidence.

Tetanus

Tetanus is caused by the action of tetanus toxin which occurs as a result of infection by *Clostridium tetani*. Tetanus spores are present throughout the environment in soil and manure. Any wound or burn can introduce the bacterium which grow anaerobically at the wound site and thorough cleaning must be undertaken of all wounds. A number of factors have been identified which increase the risk of infection occurring:

- Wounds which involve a significant amount of devitalized tissue
- Puncture wounds: especially if contaminated with soil or manure
- Wounds which require surgical intervention which is delayed for >6 hours
- Wounds with FBs in situ
- Compound fractures
- Wounds occurring in patients with systemic sepsis

Any wound fulfilling the above criteria may be considered high risk if it is heavily contaminated with material likely to carry tetanus spores, or if a large amount of devitalized tissue is present. In theses cases human tetanus immunoglobulin will be required regardless of previous vaccination.

The incubation period for the disease is between 4–21 days. Tetanus manifests itself with muscle stiffness, often in the jaw (lockjaw) and the neck which then becomes more generalized with rigidity and muscle spasms developing. It is a notifiable disease in the UK.[1]

:☠: Major haemorrhage

Major haemorrhage is a life-threatening emergency and is often associated with multiple trauma although it can occur with isolated injury to major vessels. Patients require immediate senior medical review and the attention of a trauma team if available. A full primary and secondary survey must be performed as it is easy to be distracted by the obvious wound and therefore to miss other potentially serious injuries.

Key signs and symptoms
- Obvious bleeding wound
- Tachypnoea
- Tachycardia
- Pallor

Key observations and findings
- Vital signs will require constant monitoring

Key investigations
- Bloods for U&E, FBC, cross match
- None required initially

Key actions and treatment
- As with all major trauma, a full primary survey should be completed
- Urgent senior medical review
- High-flow O_2 via a non-rebreathing mask
- Direct wound pressure and limb elevation if appropriate
- IV access × 2: large-bore cannulae if possible
- IV fluids if BP and pulse are stable
- O negative blood if tachycardia and hypotension are present
- Patients who are hypotensive or shocked require urgent surgery to locate and stop the bleeding

📖 See Major trauma, p.293.

☢ Gunshot wounds

The damage caused by a gunshot wound is related to the type of weapon, the ammunition used, the distance from the weapon and the part of the body hit. The major component of this is the velocity of the weapon. The higher the velocity, the more kinetic energy the bullet carries. A high-velocity weapon such as a rifle will create a temporary cavity up to 300 times larger than the bullet itself causing tissue and organ damage some distance from the apparent wound tract. A low velocity weapon such as a handgun is more likely just to damage the tissue it passes through. Entrance wounds are usually small and unremarkable whereas exit wounds are usually more severe.

If police are not already aware of a gunshot incident they must be informed immediately under UK firearms legislation. The patient's consent is *not* required for this. Police will require the patient's clothing for forensic investigation. Each item must be handled with gloves and placed in a separate individual paper bag which has been labelled with the patient's details and names of all staff who have handled it. The tops of the bags should be folded over and not stuck or stapled down.

As for all major trauma, a full primary and secondary survey is required along with early involvement of a senior clinician.

📖 See Major trauma, p.293.

☢ Stab wounds

Stab wounds are the most common type of penetrating injuries in the UK, usually resulting from assault. If the weapon has been removed, the resulting entry wound may look innocuous despite significant injuries to underlying structures. If the weapon is still present do not attempt to remove it. In cases of assault the police must be informed. Patient's clothing should be preserved in the same manner as for gunshot wounds. Treatment should follow the principles of ATLS with a full primary and secondary survey being undertaken along with early involvement of a senior clinician.

📖 See Major trauma, p.293.

ⓘ Minor haemorrhage

Minor haemorrhage can usually be controlled by direct pressure and elevation. Tourniquets should not be used to stop the bleeding except as a temporary measure to provide a bloodless field while the wound is explored. They should always be clamped, never tied. Calcium alginates dressings may be used to assist in achieving haemostasis. Minor haemorrhage should not cause cardiovascular instability. Any abnormalities in vital signs should trigger a further assessment. All patients should be asked to lie down prior to wound assessment due to the risk of fainting. Once the haemorrhage has been controlled the wounds should be examined, cleaned, closed, and dressed as appropriate.

Further reading

1. Department of Health (2008). *Immunisation against Infectious disease–The Green Book 2008.* London: DH.

Index